CW00816191

TRAINING THE HORSE IN HAND

TRAINING THE HORSE IN HAND

The classical Iberian principles

Alfons J. Dietz

Cadmos Verlag GmbH Brunsbek
Copyright of original German edition © 2000 Cadmos Verlag
Copyright of this edition © 2004 Cadmos Verlag
Design and Layout: Ravenstein Brain Pool
Translation: Desiree Gerber
Project Management: Editmaster Co Ltd, Northampton
Cover photo and text photos: Klaus-Jürgen Guni
Photos pp.33, 91, 130, 147: Helmut Schweige;
p.17: Helga Dietz; p.88: Bernard Kreisa
Print: Westermann Druck, Zwickau, Germany
Printed in Germany

ISBN 3-86127-911-8

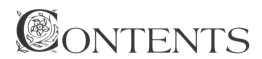CONTENTS

Foreword

My life has revolved around horses since my earliest memories, mainly due to the fact that my father and grandfather before him used to have associations with horses and also worked with them. My father, to whom I owe a vast amount of my knowledge about the art of riding and how to deal with horses, was a professional rider who bestowed all his love and attention to horses, training and caring for them. This book is dedicated to him.

In my youth, the sport of riding was taken for granted and not considered at all special. Only a great deal later, when I deliberately started to think about the training of horses, did I seriously embark on the suitable training of the living entity called the horse.

I received my early training from my father up to the age of fifteen when I joined the Spanish Riding School of Vienna. At that time the head of the riding school was the renowned Brigadier Kurt Albrecht, who is currently a dressage judge. I think there are only a few loca-

tions where, from the onset, the art of riding can be studied with such elevated excellence as in the Spanish Riding School of Vienna.

Nowhere else does one have the opportunity to accompany horses through all the phases of training, from the young, unbroken stallion right through to the completely trained horse. There is no other school that values the importance of the correct seat and the influence it has on the horse as greatly as the Rriding School in Vienna. There is hardly any other location, with the exception of the Iberian Peninsula, where training together with completion of work in hand is possible.

I stayed in the Spanish Riding School for eight years before I left to become independent and train competition horses.

It was a complete coincidence that I started to occupy myself with Iberian horses. I happened to acquire the Lusitano stallion Cartucho, whom you will often see in this book.

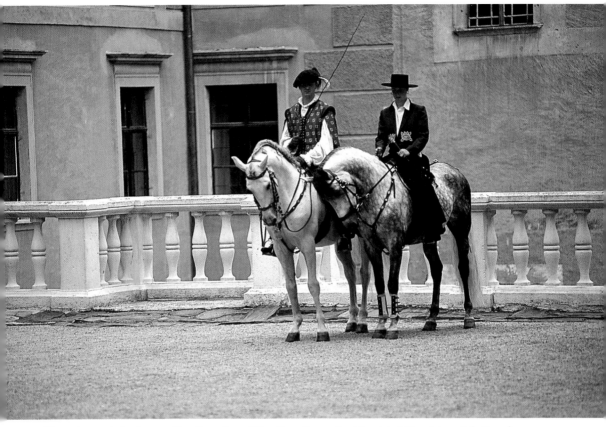

The author on the Lusitano stallion Cartucho and his wife on the purebred Spanish stallion Julepe at the Rosenburg Palace in Austria.

This horse was the incentive that took me to Portugal and Spain, where I broadened my knowledge of the art of riding at the source of its origin.

Today I work with all suitable breeds of horses, using the classical principles of the art of riding. My religion brought with it a changed attitude towards the being of the horse; I have been a Buddhist for almost ten years now and, through the philosophy that accompanies it, I have become acquainted with one of the few religions that considers all living beings equal and preaches harmony between them. The principles: "never separate your soul from love and compassion" and "the way is the goal" are never far from my work with horses today. The horse is, like you and me, a living being with similar feelings; it has strengths but also faults and weaknesses that you sometimes have to accept and forgive.

Introduction

"The art of riding", this concept is on everyone's lips, but what exactly is the art of riding? Is it an art to ride horses or an art to train horses to the highest level of education? No, the art of riding lies very much deeper than that. It starts with where I handle my horse and how considerately I handle my horse.

A sign of a talented rider is that he thinks like the horse, he knows the ways a horse thinks and reacts.

The art of riding lies in being able to understand and see through the cause and effect of everything you do. This manifests itself in the correct way of caring for and managing the horse, and the sympathetic way in which a young horse should be trained, without generating bad experiences.

The horse as a living being should be a cheerful collaborator and partner, not a disgraced object that is discarded in the corner after use: therein lies the art of managing horses and of training them successfully.

> "Ride a horse in such a way that it will be poleased with itself and want to create a proud and delightful appearance."
>
> (From "The art of riding" Xenophon)

If you abide by these rules when you work with your friend the horse, he will in return be a joyful companion that will be eager to do anything for you. What is more, the horse will most probably educate you more than you could ever wish to teach it in return: matters akin to compassionate love, sensitivity and humility. These are the most significant human virtues necessary in order to work with horses for them not to lose their grace and beauty.

It might come as a surprise in this book that I sometimes give more detailed information on the classical work with the ridden horse. The reason lies in the fact that the work in hand and the ridden work are intimately interwoven. For many movements, for example the piaffe, the work in

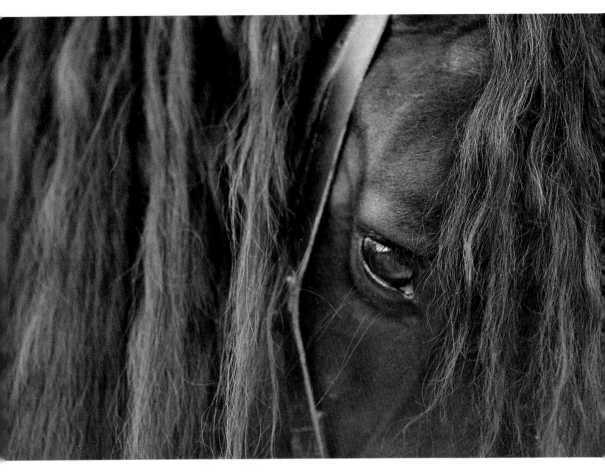

Complete trust is the first principle of the art of riding

hand depicts the supreme approach to initiate it, for others it might represent the perfect method to improve and hone the technique.

Some lessons must be taught from the saddle before the technique can be used in hand. This means that the work under the rider and the work in hand form a firm and inseparable link.

Another thing I need to say in this introduction, is that nothing written in this book is "my method", as so many so-called riding gurus claim to have developed a new technique.

There are experiences that are thousands of years old, which I have been allowed to discover in my own life and have become richer for doing so. These are not new insights into the horse, for neither man nor horse has, as far as their appearance or social conditions are concerned, changed dramatically in the last few hundred years.

Everything you read here is therefore "clinically tested" through the skill and knowledge of the old masters and myself and only written in modern words. So I wish you a tremendous amount of fun reading and applying this old wisdom.

History and Origins
of Work in Hand

Allow me to lengthen my stride even further! Work in hand as a gymnastic exercise has its origin in the antique world. The Greek Xenophon, born around 438 BC, taught a method already used by the Olympic athletes and adapted for horses. He created the first apprenticeship for riding – applicable to this day. His most famous saying was:

> *"The sense of dressage lies therein that a horse can be enabled to carry the weight of a rider up to an advanced age, without inflicting damage upon itself."*

I think we must seriously consider this sentence today. The riders of antiquity also realised that the work in hand made many lessons easier for the horse.

The centuries following such ancient times more or less put the art of riding on ice, right past the Middle Ages. It was only in the Renaissance, around the year 1670, that the skill of riding experienced new growth. This is when work in hand first came into being.

Antoine de Pluvinel, riding instructor of his majesty the king of France, is considered to be the inventor of the lunge post and the paired posts, the so-called pillars. That he was the actual inventor cannot be proven for a fact, but he was definitely the first to integrate work in hand into his way of training horses.

He left us with a written work of his techniques, the riding instructions for the king ("L'instruction du Roy"). Unfortunately, his labour had (and still has) a disad-

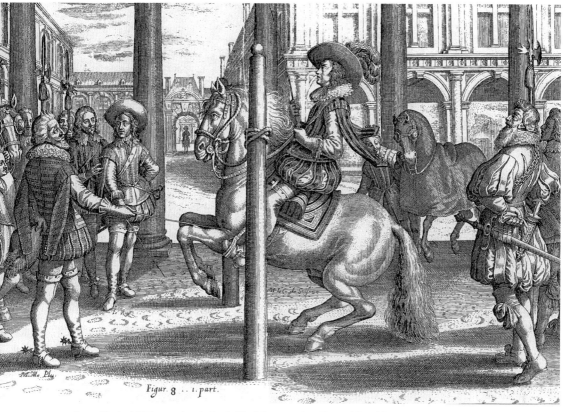

From Pluvinel "L'instruction de Roy": Work between the pillars with a rider

vantage in that it is not suitable for every horse and it can be downright dangerous if it is not used with the necessary knowledge and care. This will be examined in more detail later in this book.

At this time the training of horses still gave priority to their use in war. The contest of man against man on horseback was the centre of attention. This meant horses had to be capable of performing sharp turns and canter pirouettes, racing from standstill and sliding halts with just the slightest change in the bodyweight, for both the rider's hands were busy with the handling of weapons in the battle.

At the beginning of the eighteenth century, the art of riding became a means in itself. This was a time of supremacy for French talent. The Frenchman Francois Robichon de la Guérinière left his mark with the importance he placed on the work in hand as a means to truthful riding.

Guérinière was the first to be resolute in the matter that horses can be trained in a delicate manner in his book "Principles of French Riding". He used Pluvinel's pillars only with certain horses and worked the horses mainly free in hand, with only a cavesson, in exactly the same way the Spanish Riding School does to this day.

Some years later, a new master saw the light in the field of work in hand, namely the stable master of the Prussian Royal in Hannover. He was also successful in the use of the pillars and drew up a document, „Training the riding and carriage horse in the pillars", that gives a detailed explanation of this matter.

Mazzuchelli (1760-1830) can be described as the father of the long rein. He recor-

ded the masterpiece "Elementi de Cavalerizza" where he describes the facets of work in hand in particular. He developed the long reins, connecting two reins to the cavesson, one on the inside and one on the outside.

There are of course many more masters that practised riderless training of the horse, for example the Englishman James Fillis or the circus rider Baucher, himself a student of Mazzuchelli.

They are, however, thought of as fraudsters in classical dressage circles, for much of their basic information was interpreted incorrectly when unnatural lessons were "trained", for example the canter back-

Work on long reins with "Spanish rider", according to Mazzuchelli.

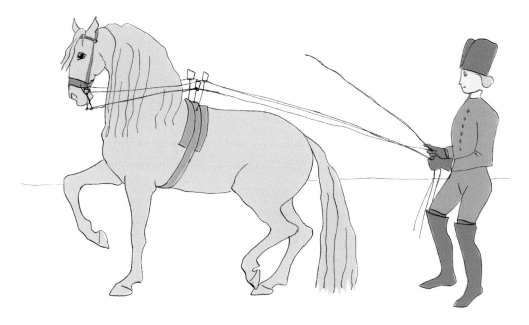

wards or piaffe on three legs. Critics of these masters, of whom there are many today, often do not think of the horses that were used in those times. In every riding apprenticeship a trainer ever tries to attempt, it is of utmost importance to consider the breed and the substance of horse that the trainer has available. Only then can one draw any conclusions from the prevailing effort.

For all the unnatural movements James Fillis expected from his horses, it has to be said that he was a sympathetic rider, for how else would it be possible to teach a horse such impertinent and unnatural things?

Physical and psychological Requirements of the Trainer and the Horse

The prerequisites for both horse and rider to be engaged in the work in hand have a physical as well as a psychological nature.

The ideal trainer, seen from a psychological point of view, is a thinking, sympathetic person with a good eye for movement and no tendency to lose his temper and punish the horse unjustly. The ideal trainer is therefore of constant and steadfast character. The physical side is as important for the work in hand cannot be separated from the work in the saddle. The trainer will thus require an excellent and correct seat, the base on which classical riding is built.

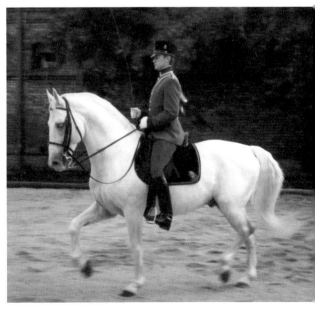

The correct classical-modern seat.

It is no small wonder that the Spanish Riding School of Vienna maintains a strong view on the development of a proficient seat. The riders that join the school spend several years training their seat on the lunge.

THE CORRECT SEAT OF THE RIDER

Imagine you have a little monkey of about 20 kilograms that you carry in a backpack. The monkey pulls and strains to the left in the bag while you try to go to the right. If you are trained in this way of going, it will be at the very least unpleasant. If you are not trained in this way of going, you will find it close to impossible to move in the desired direction. This and worse is how our horses feel when an uncoordinated and untrained rider tries to ride. How often do we see a rider that wants to do a half-pass to the left, but meanwhile hangs over to the right, thus preventing the horse from moving in the correct direction? To top it all, the horse will also be reprimanded for not doing the "right" thing!

The seat of the rider has changed and been improved upon, always according to the requirements of the relevant period of history. The seat in the Renaissance, for example, was completely different from that we use today. At this time people still fought on horseback. Competition between knights with lances was at that time custo-

mary. For this reason the riders of the Renaissance used the fork seat with the legs stretched far to the front. This gave valuable support: you could sturdily bear weight on the stirrups while at the same time lean back forcefully into the high cantles of the saddles of those times.

In baroque times the lance seat became unfashionable, and the seat changed again. The leg shifted to the back, but was still, in comparison with today, in an extremely long position. Riding became an art form and the horse a continuation of the rider. Elegance was of the utmost importance, hence the too long leg in the stirrup and the excessively short upper body that we see so often in the paintings of the aristocracy of the period. Everything was exaggerated and romanticised in this era, it was simply the epoch of fine art.

The seat as we know it today, serves a particular purpose, is effective from the point of view of the rider, gentle on the horse and to top it all is elegant and looks proficient. This seat came into being in the era of classicism, the military period in the 19th century. This change in the seat of the rider was also brought about by practical requirements at the time. Now the rider had to have a seat that enabled jumping over obstacles on horseback. The stirrup leathers became shorter (the stirrups became used more specifically to stand in) and the posture became more upright, with slight tension and strongly bent ankles. The classical school seat was born!

In detail the classical seat comprises the following:

The head is in an upright position and follows the direction of movement of the horse. Both the shoulders should be held in a relaxed way, pulled back somewhat and always parallel to the shoulders of the horse (see lateral movements). The upper arms lie loosely against the body, the fore-arm and hand give the appearance of being in a straight line to the horse's mouth via the reins. In an ideal world the hands will be approximately one hand's breadth above the horse's withers, carried lightly, as if holding two glasses of water. The back must be straight, without hollowing and without any tension. The hips should be held parallel to the hips of the horse and must swing lightly and rhythmically to the movement of the horse's hips, without interfering with the natural sequence. The leg of the rider must be bent somewhat and must be positioned flat from the hips. This way it will be placed quietly with a flat calf against the horse. The ankle is pushed low down and with every step of the trot it must swing down even deeper. Head, shoulder, hip and ankle must give rise to a straight line.

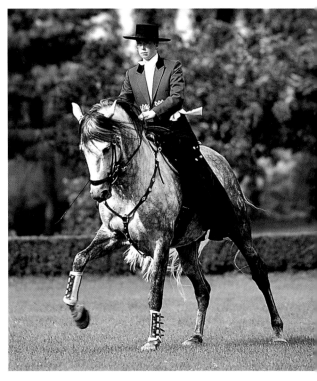

The same rule applies in the Iberian school: if the seat is not correct, the desired results cannot be achieved.

PHYSICS OF RIDING

The implementation of the rider's seat may have several irreversible effects and specific limitations that arise from the anatomy of the rider and the horse and can only be explained on a physical level.

Here are a few examples to clarify what I mean by that statement:

The head of the rider has a not insignificant weight in comparison to the body, which makes it important for the rider to look in the direction of the movement. If the head is turned shortly before the horse has to turn, it often works a treat! The same applies for the shoulders, which should be held parallel to the shoulders of the horse and in this way assist the horse to step under the weight of the rider in the lateral gaits and on the turns.

This brings us neatly to the significance of the rider's weight. When more weight is placed on the stirrups at the same time as the seat bones of the rider are burdened, the horse will automatically step in the appropriate direction, in other words, under the weight of the rider.

This will often bring disagreement for example with the western riding style, where in some lessons the horse is frequently taught to react to weight signals that are quite the opposite of what is taught in the classical style. Clearly a horse can be taught just about anything, even that the command for the canter on the right lead is "sausage". This is no more than a bogus way of riding. A horse is conditioned by the repetition of a command. This cannot be classified as art or as athletic ability.

The dynamic force of the rider's hips produces the power of the seat that propels the horse, similar to the tipping of a stool with the seat. (Try the stool trick for a better understanding of the function of driving hips). The easiest way to produce a half-halt with the seat is simply to breathe out deeply, let the hand become quiet after a few half-halts and apply slight leg pressure. This is a lesson that is easily tested from the canter transition into the trot; even young horses will do it without so much as batting an eyelid. The weight of the rider that moves forward a little will have a decelerating effect on the horse.
This is easily illustrated when observing a beginner on horseback. They swing to and fro in a typically uncoordinated fashion. The effect this oscillation has on the horse cannot be ignored. The rider's upper body moves to the front and the horse slows down, this will abruptly be rectified by a kick from the legs at which the horse will react by going forwards. All these contradictory aids from the rider are naturally somewhat startling to the horse and that can lead to total confusion. As the horse is moving forward and the unbalanced rider falls behind the vertical line, the movement functions as double dynamic and the horse all but runs away from it. In the futile attempt to do the right thing, the poor horse gets jerked in the mouth by the rider's hands and the situation starts all over again.

As you can see, there are certain unchangeable effects that the rider has on the horse. Maybe it is at this point that it becomes easy to understand the merit of a sound classical seat, the basic requirement of an accomplished rider.

CONFORMATION AND TEMPERAMENT OF THE HORSE

The psychological prerequisites for working in hand are more or less the same for the horse as for the human training it. The main characteristic sought after will be an honest horse with no demanding dominant behaviour, such as found often in thoroughbred stallions.

I will go into more detail of the different characteristics of the breeds that are specific for the work in hand a little later. For the moment I want to pay particular attention to the various types of horses and their physical advantages and weaknesses when particularly looking for horses for work in hand.

THE SQUARE HORSE

As can be concluded from the heading, this is a horse in the square configuration. In this type of horse the measurement from point of shoulder to the point of buttock is equal to the height of the horse up to the withers. The biggest advantage of this type of horse is that it is capable of a great deal of collection. This is based on the fact that the hindquarters can effortlessly be brought closer to the forehand, enabling weight to be carried on the hindquarters more easily. This type of horse will show exceptional capabilities in the more collected movements such as piaffe, passage and canter pirouette. Unfortunately it does not always have the capacity for big range and thus only shows an average talent for extended gaits such as medium trot and medium canter. Andalusians, Lusitanos and Lipizzaners are typical square types.

THE RECTANGULAR HORSE

Most sporting horses can at the present time be classified as rectangular types. The biggest

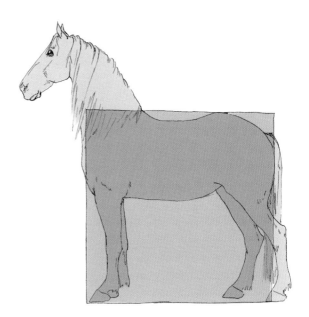

The square horse

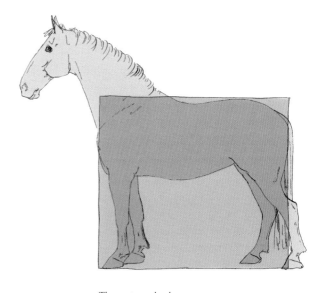

The rectangular horse

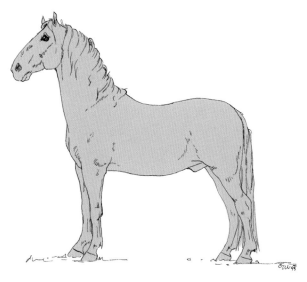

Correct conformation for a horse

advantage these horses have is their enormous length of stride. Horses with longer backs are normally capable of taking longer strides. Most of these horses are capable of only average collection but have the bigger flashy strides of the extended trot and extended canter and even long strides in the walk that are much in demand in today's sport horse.

Collection in these horses can be immensely increased with work in hand. This must, however, be performed slowly and with great care, for they must be taught to pick themselves up to go into collection.

CONFORMATION – STRENGTHS AND WEAKNESSES

Let us start on the hindquarters, for we work our horses from behind to become soft over the back up into the poll.

In this region there is an essential and important prerequisite to observe, namely the angle of the stifle and hock joints, for these can make the effort of training more or less demanding. A too open stifle joint, meaning the angle is too big, can be a difficult situation in training. Sickle hocks, where the angle of the hocks is too dramatic, can also be a drawback. It is furthermore important to carry out the necessary power training of the muscles in order to avoid undue strain on the joints and to enable the joints to withstand the extra bending demanded in collection. At first sight the dock of the tail can say a great deal about the quality of the hindquarters: a high set tail suggests a middle-of-the-road ability towards collection, a lower set tail implies a superior talent for collection.

The connection of the croup to the back is enormously important: a strong and direct connection will indicate that the power generated in the hindquarters can be converted into power to carry the horse, in other words it is the criterion of the carrying capacity. In an ideal world the horse carries at least two thirds of its body weight on the hindquarters. A weak link in the croup will show all the signs of hardship as far as carrying capacity goes. Special attention should be given to the back of the horse, for this is after all the space where we sit. A correctly fitting saddle as a matter of course and well developed musculature is desired. The back should be wide and well muscled but not too long in comparison to the height of the horse.

A decent angle of the forehand will cause the movements to appear light and graceful and will have a positive effect on the ground covering aspect. Horses with a more upright shoulder will move somewhat stiffly with little movement in the shoulder and the rider will sit with more restriction.

The natural way the neck is attached to the body is a decisive factor for that will determine the foundation of the topline of the horse. This means the high set in the shoulder of the baroque horse is the epitome of a dressage horse. The neck should not look as if "stuck on" the horse, but should have a flowing line out of the shoulder. The way the neck is set should be neither too strong (like that of a bull) nor too weak (having a degenerated look). The jowl should have enough freedom and not obstruct the bend in the horse's head and neck.

The mouth of the horse is more often than not given too much thought, for we only have to ride the horse from behind into the bit and not the other way round. There are, however, some arguments for looking at the horse's mouth, for the form will determine the type of bit we need to use. An important condition is the height and undulation of the palate of the mouth. In a flat palate any kind of bit that allows space for the tongue or even a plain snaffle will involuntarily pierce into the palate and may even injure it. Palpation will soon

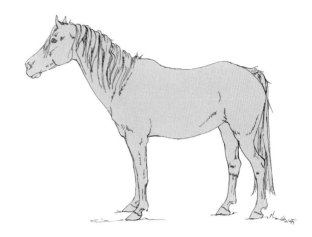

Faulty conformation: a too deep-set neck, upright shoulder and hocks.

reveal an almost square (and more sensitive) mouth or a rounder (less sensitive) mouth. If the horse is a stallion or a gelding, the position of the canine teeth must also be considered. Individual taste, sometimes in the real sense of the word, will determine the choice of material (for example stainless steel, copper, rubber).

THE INFLUENCE OF TEMPERAMENT ON TRAINING

The character of the horse will have a considerable influence on the training, and in most cases will almost be more important that the conformation of the horse. In this way I have seen many horses make up for their physical faults by sheer determination and intelligent trainability. On the other side of the coin one can often find horses with virtually perfect conformation that are entirely unsuitable to be trained in the classical system, purely because of their disposition.

In order to do proper work in hand, a horse with a medium to strong, but nevertheless obedient temperament is sought.

Horses with explosive and unpredictable temperaments, or those that have been spoilt by human contact are not, if truth be told, suitable for the job. On the other hand, these horses can benefit the most from the correct work in hand by someone who is familiar with the techniques. The main prerequisite for these horses is that they must still, after all that has been done to them, be honest. Horses that are notorious for kicking and rearing are only corrected in the exception and not as the rule.

Basic Principles
of the Art of
Riding

Before we fully turn our attention to the work in hand, we need to clarify certain basic principles of the art of riding that are also applicable to the work we want to do in hand.

The goal of riding is ultimately to train a horse to be agile, calm, and obedient and to have agreeable movement. The physical effort of working with such a horse is not taxing, but full of lightness, the so-called "légéreté" as it is called by the French. I often heard the trainers in the Spanish Riding School in Vienna say to me: "Always stay light!" This is relevant to all horses, regardless of whether they are trained for jumping, dressage or hacking, and even more so for the horses that do practical labour such as those of the Spanish and Portuguese cowboys and mounted matadors, the "rejoneador".

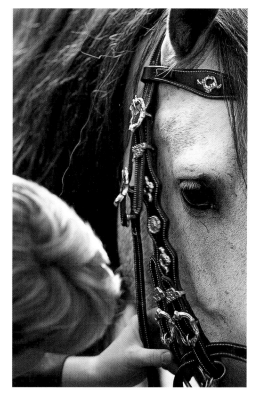

Inspecting the bridle before riding is essential.

To make sure that you are on the right track, you have to assess your horse's progress from time to time using the basic principles of riding.

In the Spanish Riding School the old-fashioned term "lesson" is used for the daily work with the horse. This daily exertion is divided into repetitions of differing lengths that are always interspersed by phases of relaxation and complete calm in order not to overtax the horse. The horse should not be worn-out first before an attempt is made to teach it something new, but the available energy must rather be channelled into the positive route of education. In other words, the steps the horse makes at the end of a lesson should be as vivacious as the ones at the start of the lesson. It is enormously important that the lesson should terminate before the horse shows any signs of weakness! We must capitalise on the excellent memory of the horse by concluding a well-executed lesson on a high level with abundant praise and ushering the horse back to its stable or paddock. On no account may the horse end a lesson on a negative note, for the horse will come out of the stable the next day in exactly the same mood it was returned there: annoyed or pleased to work.

As soon as a horse commences to follow a lesson and even think ahead by anticipating the aids of the rider, it is always a good sign – the horse is in fact pleased to work! Such a horse must never be punished. The horse must yet learn to follow the lesson on the rider's command, and this is the reason for incorporating many changes of pace, direction and chronological order into the lesson.

Apart from a proficient knowledge of psychology and physiology, it is equally important to possess a concept of the movement and centre of gravity of the horse. Theory cannot replace experience, but knowledge should always precede actions!

BASIC GAITS AND THOSE OF HIGH SCHOOL MOVEMENTS

The uncomplicated, natural gaits are walk, trot and canter, whereas the high school gaits include lateral gaits, piaffe, passage and rein back. Gaits are distinguished according to the sequence of the footfalls in the movement. The tempo is the distance covered in a specific time, in which the rhythm – the repeated and consistent placing of the foot – should not change. Cadence is the increased liveliness and setting down of the feet. Stronger cadence is seen in the development of improved collection. The higher steps of a nervous horse, however, must not be mistaken for cadence. These nervous steps are mostly a sign of tension in the topline of the horse. Rhythm and cadence do not have the same meaning either, even though it may seem that way in the beginning. A rigid and inexpressive horse can trot with rhythm without showing any signs of cadence. On the other hand, cadence without rhythm is not possible. The expression of the trot is lost without rhythm and becomes tainted.

The use of a metronome is recommended to ensure and review the purity of the rhythm and cadence. The individual rhythm of a horse can be revealed with the help of a video camera where the steps are counted per minute. The metronome can now be adjusted to this specific rhythm and the horse can be worked in hand or under a rider according to this beat. With a higher degree of training and more collection or in the piaffe and passage the horse will step with more cadence. The expression of the horse will often make a surprising transformation as soon as the rhythm or cadence is changed. If you have a piece of music that is in rhythm with your horse, it can constitute a pleasant substitute for the metronome. However, if you want to make use of a metronome, you should be able to buy one readily from a music store. Metronomes are available in small sizes similar to a pocket watch that can be secured on your collar or coat.

WALK

At the walk, the feet of the horse are placed one after the other on the ground, making four audible beats : left foreleg, right hindleg, right foreleg, left hindleg. The uppermost principle of the walk: same side but not at the same time!

In the walk there is no moment of suspension, in other words there are always two or three legs on the ground at any given time. Any change in the rhythm of the walk will jeopardise the purity of the gait and could lead to unwanted pacing. The hurrying of the walk is as incorrect as pacing even if the horse stays in the correct footfall sequence of the walk. The sequence of the walk does not change in the medium, collected or free walk; only the length and grandeur of the stride will change. In the medium and free walk the hindfeet must overstep the imprint of the forefeet, whereas it is not required in the collected walk and it is even acceptable for the imprint of the hindfoot to be a full hoof print behind that of the forefoot. In training the normal walk is preferred to the collected walk, which is not used frequently in order not to jeopardise the sequence of the walk. The horse should stride out in the walk, which is in the truest sense what the walk is all about.

TROT

The trot is a natural two-beat pace on alternate diagonal legs: left hindleg and right foreleg, moment of suspension, right hindleg and left foreleg, moment of suspension. The horse carries his own weight and should the need arise, that of the rider on the two legs of the diagonal pairs. As in the walk, the footfall sequence of the trot remains completely independent of the tempo.

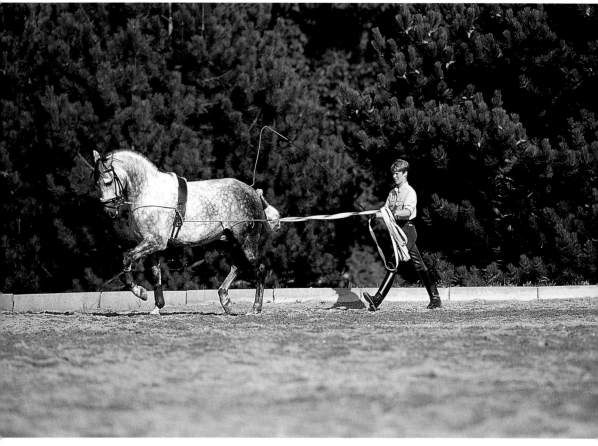

Julepe in forward trot

If the tempo is reduced, the moment of suspension is also shortened. If the pace is intensified, the length of the stride will increase into a more extended trot and the moment of suspension will also be prolonged.

In the collected trot, the horse will spend more time on the diagonal legs as a form of support. At the same time the horse will lift its legs higher and it is these splendid, rhythmical and energetic steps that are described as cadenced. As is the case with the walk, in the collected steps of the trot the footprints of the hindlegs do not step into those left by the forelegs but stay well back. In the working trot the hindfoot will step into the print of the forefoot, whereas in the medium and extended trots the hindfoot will overstep the prints of the forefoot. The legs of the horse will reach their utmost in the extended trot.

It is considered a defect when a horse forges, audible especially in the extended trot. This happens when the toe of the hindfoot strikes the forefoot and a metallic clicking can be heard. The front leg of the horse remains on the ground too long and the hindleg then "overtakes" the foreleg. This indicates that the horse is on the forehand and the result is often that shoes are lost. The remedy is to shorten the stride length and ask the horse to lift more in the front.

An extended trot that shows a spectacular scope with the front legs but unmatched hindleg movement must be considered faulty. In this case the hindquarters must drive the back legs to match the front legs by stepping more under the body of the horse.

The trot is generally considered to be the most important basic gait in the training of the horse. Any faults that slip in here will have an effect on the other basic gaits.

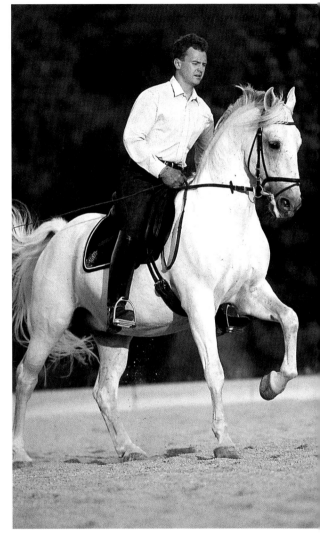

Canter is a jumping motion in three beats

CANTER

Canter is in essence a jumping motion where three obvious beats are heard: outside hindleg, inside hindleg and outside foreleg, outside foreleg, moment of suspension. The difference between canter and the other two basic gaits is that the canter has a right and left option, depending on which foreleg is in the lead. There are one, two and three legged support phases where the horse carries his weight and that of the rider on one or all of these legs. As in the other gaits the sequence of the footfalls stays the same, regardless of the tempo.

Like the trot, the canter has four tempi: collected canter, working canter, medium canter and extended canter. In addition, the gallop can be added where the most coverage of ground is made. This was used in the cavalry attacks in the previous centuries and is only seen in horse racing nowadays. The correct canter is an active jumping movement where the horse bounces like a rubber ball with an abundance of suspension from one stride to the next.

A canter is classified as faulty when four beats can be heard. This happens when the inside hindleg touches the ground earlier than the outside foreleg in the two-legged support phase. This fault arises when the tempo is shortened without the aid of the rider's legs, which means it only ensues with the aid of the reins. The result is the loss of the dynamic swing and the canter is no longer impressive. This is the single biggest fault in the canter. Another fault in the canter is the so-called disunited canter, where the horse will for example canter to the left at the back and to the right at the front. This fault will mainly occur in horses that do not yet have sufficient strength and find it hard to carry themselves in proper balance. There is also the "wrong" canter, whereby the horse will canter right on the left rein and left on the right rein. However, if this was done intentionally, it is called the counter canter. This is not to be confused with the renvers canter for it differs in that the horse canters on two tracks.

REIN BACK

The rein back is a similar movement to the trot, the horse moves backwards on the diagonal pairs of legs without a moment of suspension. If the rein back has four beats as is the case in the walk it is considered faulty. The rein back is a sign of obedience and suppleness of the horse. It should be executed readily, but not rapidly, in a good frame without dragging the feet.

PIAFFE

The piaffe is a trot on the spot with the most cadence. It has the same sequence of footfalls as the trot, but the moment of suspension is no longer than a fraction of a second. If the moment of suspension is not there, the piaffe will appear expressionless and incorrect. In the perfect piaffe, the horse will lift its fore leg almost to the horizontal and the hoof of the back leg will at the same time lift up to the fetlock joint of the supporting leg. The piaffe is regarded as faulty when the diagonal legs do not step together in their rhythm or the front feet lift high and the hindlegs stay trapped on the ground. An inability of the hindlegs to come off the ground makes it impossible for the horse to move into the trot and that in turn will trigger poor transitions. Another fault in the piaffe is when the legs cross over when executing the movement.

The piaffe is a learnt gait, but it is seen in nature. In nature the horse will do a piaffe when it feels threatened and pushed into a corner. The forward movement is prevented and the horse will trot on the spot. As soon as the obstruction is removed, the horse will immediately move forward ata trot.

PASSAGE

In old books the passage is also called the Spanish step. In the passage the horse will spring onto the diagonal pair of legs and hold, depending on the build of its body, the elevated legs for longer and higher than in the normal trot. The moment of suspension is prolonged the most in the passage. In an ideal passage the impression is created of floating free from gravity.

The passage requires a strong, gymnastic horse that is able to maintain his balance without any tension. If this is not the case, it will seem as if the hindlegs do not step under the horse's centre of gravity and therefore carry very little weight. The following faults can result from this:

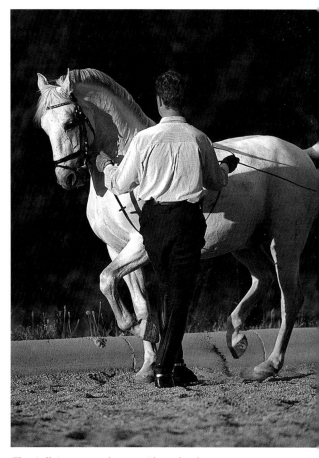

The piaffe is a trot on the spot with an abundance of cadence

- · Too short a moment of suspension: the horse cannot carry its own weight and then steps too fast.
- · Irregular steps: the horse will lift one hindleg higher than the other – in the Spanish Riding School this is called "kicking".
- · Swaying in the passage: the horse sways in the movement and seen from the front the legs will cross over.

- · It is also incorrect to classify a floating trot as passage. This is only a manife station of tension the horse is trying to conquer.

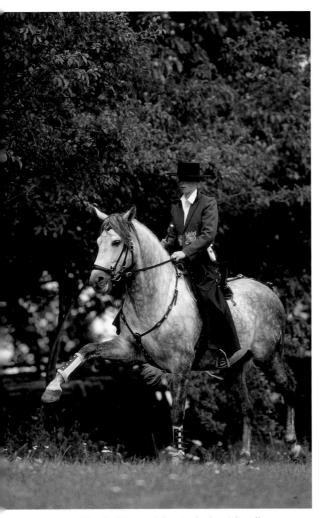

Claudia Dietz on Julepe in the Spanish walk

all too easily be lost. Teaching a horse the sequence of the movements, even though they are natural, without the accepted preparation, is foolishness and has nothing to do with athletic ability.

THE SPANISH WALK

The Spanish walk is very popular on the Iberian Peninsula, mainly owing to the spectacular effect it has. This movement is not categorised in the classical vocabulary, for it is generally held that the horse will not step beyond the plumb line that is created from the nostrils to the ground. However, if you observe young stallions in the paddock, you will notice that this guideline is not accurate, for in their mock fights the colts will strike out with their front legs way in front of this plumb line. From this particular method of mock fighting between stallions the Spanish walk is derived. In the Spanish walk the sequence of the footfalls in the walk is retained. The walk is to some extent collected and ideally the leg is raised to an almost horizontal line, without intrusion on the rhythm. The Spanish walk is flawed when the hindlegs do not follow through. This shortcoming will hinder the flow of the movement, for the horse will take bigger steps in front and smaller ones behind. It is equally faulty when the front legs pound the ground: the horse should gently place the foreleg on the ground, only then can the Spanish walk be breathtaking.

Unfortunately, because it is visually such an impressive movement, the trend today is to expect a passage too early in the horse's education. I would strongly advise against that. This movement should only follow the systematic training of the correct muscles, for the "classical passage" can

PARAMETERS OF TRAINING

In this section certain parameters of training that are also applicable to the work in hand will be elaborated upon. This is not a matter of stringing together some goals in the training process that can be achieved one after the other, but rather a kind of curriculum, where each element can only function in relation to all the others.

THE HORSE IN BALANCE

Unfortunately, very few horses have a natural ability for dance-like skills. Like their human counterparts, they have to learn to move in balance with themselves, especially as they do not only have to carry just their own weight, but also that of the rider in balance.

In contrast to the human, a horse does not carry his weight on two legs where the centre of gravity is almost directly above,

THE PYRAMID
OF CLASSICAL TRAINING

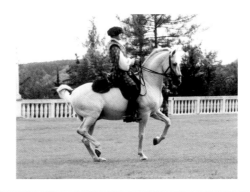

The objective	**THE OBJECTIVE COLLECTION**
	PLIABILITY (DURCHLÄSSIGKEIT)
The building bricks	**THE BUILDING BRICKS STRAIGHTNESS AND SUPPLENESS**
	IMPULSION(SCHWUNG)
	CONTACT
	REGULARITY AND BALANCE
The Foundation	**THE FOUNDATION RELAXATION**

but on four legs, which changes the perspective completely. If the rider does not ride the horse in a correct manner, the horse's weight will move more to the forehand. From an anatomical point of view, the front legs are not suitable for carrying weight but for support only; the result is that the horse is not in balance. Balance is the basic prerequisite for a rhythmical and supple way of moving.

As soon as a rider enters the equation it becomes more complicated. The centre of gravity for both the horse and rider must be taken into account if the horse is not to be prevented from correctly moving forwards. If you have ever had the opportunity to ride a young horse, you will have experienced the initial clumsiness of the horse, which stems from the unusual burden of the rider's weight that confuses the horse's sense of balance. Very few horses are naturally balanced or find being ridden relatively unproblematic. Owing to this lack of balance the sense of "lightness" will be absent in the beginning. In the continuous training of the horse, this lightness is promoted by the hindquarters stepping further under the body, thus building up the weight–carrying capacity in the hindlegs.

> *Balance is the basic prerequisite for a rhythmical and supple way of moving.*

CONTACT

Contact can be described as the light connection the horse has on his lips with the bit. It is an elastic bond between the rider's hand and the horse's mouth that comes from accepting the bit. This connection facilitates guiding and collection of the horse and can only come about when the horse is soft and giving in the neck and if the rider's hand reacts in a correspondingly sensitive fashion. Complete contact is only then possible when the horse does not use the hand of the rider to lean against, but stays entirely balanced in his own centre of gravity. Balance and the acceptance of the bit influence each other mutually: the contact on the bit will for example be of higher quality in an older horse that is balanced than in a young horse, and vice versa. A horse with true contact will find its balance superior to that of a horse with difficulty in accepting the bit.

Contact depends on a number of factors: the build of the horse's body, the horse's temperament and the nature of the horse's mouth will all play significant roles.

A horse with weak hindquarters will show a tenacious contact that leads to the horse leaning on the reins, for this horse will try to evade the possibility of being overtaxed when the hindquarters start to engage. In a case like this, taking up more reins or giving slack with the rein will have absolutely no influence on the horse. A wide-ranging tightness arises from general tension in the body or incorrect train-

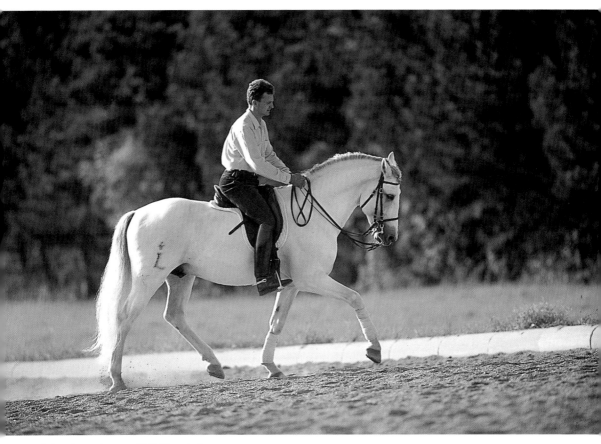

Relaxed warming up with light contact

ing that has left the mouth insensitive. Driving the hindquarters under the body and releasing and taking up of the reins by the rider can rectify this obstinate acceptance of the bit. This kind of correction is possible only to a certain degree in an apathetic horse.

There are two potential tactics a horse can use to try to resist the contact. It can either go "above the bit" where the head is noticeably in front of the vertical, or "behind the bit" where the nose disappears behind the vertical. The first problem is often seen in horses with weak backs and the second in nervous horses and horses with sensitive mouths.

Both the above-mentioned scenarios are considered faults and must receive appropriare attention. If the back proves to be weak, the horse's musculature should be allowed more time to develop, another sphere where the work in hand can come in useful and provide invaluable support. At the beginning the horse must be worked and ridden with a long neck and rounded back, the so-called "long and low" position, and gradually be raised from behind to carry itself in the correct posture and contact. If the horse is inclined to carry itself behind the bit, great care must be taken not to collect the horse too early and to guide it with a soft hand. There is also a third fault, which is the unstable contact and is especially visible in temperamental horses. The horse will switch from being above the bit to being behind the bit and back. Rectifying can be achieved by keeping the hand soft and quiet and calmly urging the horse forward.

Bearing in mind all of the above problems, there is hardly a horse that will have equal contact on both reins. This phenomenon is comparable to people who are left- or right-handed; it is a concept that might be improved, but not necessarily rectified. The basic rule: pressure will evoke pressure is applicable. If you pull on the right rein, the horse will pull on the right rein as well. Change of direction, in which you often change the rein and work a little on the "bad rein" may be of some aid: the horse must almost not notice that it is going on the bad rein. The contact will become better as the horse becomes more educated.

> *The rider does not seek the contact with the horse's mouth; the horse seeks the contact with the rider's hands!*

STRAIGHTNESS

Balance and collection is only possible when the horse is straight.

Horses will have a tendency to go crooked under a rider's weight or with false collection, especially in the school. If the horse is straightened, the hindfeet will follow exactly in the tracks of the forefeet. If the feet follow to the side it means the horse is going crooked.

In order to appreciate why a horse will go crooked, particularly in the beginning of training, you must remember that the shoulders of the horse are narrower than the hindquarters. As soon as the horse moves with its shoulders too close to the edge of the school, the inevitable outcome is that it will move in a crooked way. It is principally observed that young horses want to move with their shoulders and hindquarters the same distance from the side of the school. Many of them will even try to touch the wall with their shoulders in order to use it as a support when asked to halt on a straight line.

Correction for this is to adjust the shoulder in correlation to the hindquarters, suggesting that the shoulder come into the school more and working increasingly away from the wall and on circles.

This brings us to one of the most important rules of riding:

> *Straighten your horse*
> *and ride it forwards!*

PLIABILITY (DURCHLÄSSIGKEIT)

This term is of utmost importance in the art of riding. The horse is considered as pliable when the effect of the rein affects the body of the horse through the poll and neck, continues through the back of the horse and manifests itself in a loaded and flexed hindfoot at the same time. In order for this to function, the horse must be in the correct contact. The horse steps with its hindlegs under its supple back into the flexible hand of the rider. If the feeling in the hand is too strong, the effect of the reins cannot flow through the body of the horse but will end in the withers. If, on the other hand, there is not enough feeling in the rider's hand, the effect of the reins will end immediately in the neck or jowl. If the contact is one-sided the effect will be lost on the opposite side of the contact.

> *Durchlässigkeit is achieved when the aids*
> *are correctly and promptly executed and the*
> *prevailing rein-aid is continued to the loaded*
> *and flexed hindfoot of the same side.*

HEAD CARRIAGE

Head carriage of the horse is always the result of true contact. Head carriage in connection with the position of the neck is of fundamental importance in the gymnastic training of the horse. On the one hand the head carriage is dependent on the degree of training and on the other hand on the tempo in which the horse is worked.

Difficulty in achieving the right elevation can result from the exterior qualities of the horse. Horses with overdeveloped neck muscles or little space in the groove behind the jowl, might only be able to achieve correct head carriage after meticulous rebuilding of the muscles.

On straight lines the position of the head and neck of the horse will correspond with the straight line, on curved lines the midline of the horse must tally with the curve we are riding, which means the whole length of the horse's body is curved. When the rider looks down, the eyelashes of the inner eye must be seen. The horse must not only be soft and giving where the head goes over into the neck, but also where the neck goes over into the shoulder. This is the only way in which the correct head carriage can be achieved.

In the arena the head carriage will be slightly to the inside of the school, the only exception being the lengthened trot. In this instance it is more appropriate to position the horse as straight as possible, for any curve might bring about uneven steps and an irregular rhythm.

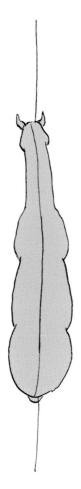

Head carriage on a straight line

The head carriage must never be achieved through pulling on the reins for the result will only be a horse that presses its neck into the shoulders.

The horse can only attain the exact head carriage when it totally accepts the bit and is ridden forward in harmonious balance with engagement in the hindquarters.

> *Head carriage is only a small portion in the development of the art of riding.*

BEND

In order to make the horse more supple and, more importantly, to stay supple and to prevent any stiffness from setting in, we have to bend the horse. In principle there are two ways of bending a horse: sideways and lengthways. Let us commence with what should be the easier method of bending for the horse in the beginning, namely sideways bending. Sideways bending incorporates the whole body of the horse, an even bend from the poll right through to the tail. As the rump curves to the outside, the ribs on the inside are somewhat compressed. In the sideways bend, it is expected that the horse bends around the inside leg of the rider and it is only required in movement. There are a few exceptions to this rule where young horses have to be taught this by bending whilst standing. The natural arch of its ribcage will determine the maximum bend of a horse.

There are different grades of this sideways bend, for example on circles, changes in direction and voltes, always keeping in mind that the midline of the horse should stay on the identical line that we ride upon. In the ideal case the horse will step lithely with its centre of gravity supported and at the same time controlling its balance in each change of direction.

All horse have a better and a worse rein. On the better rein one will often speak of a hollow ribcage: the horse will show more of a bend on this side, even occasionally too much of a bend.

Exaggerated bending should be avoided at all cost for it normally originates from the neck. The horse is in the correct bend when the neck does not bend more than the rest of the body, when it releases the jowls and is balanced in a curve. Whereas many horses exaggerate the bend to one side, they will frequently stiffen their bodies to the "worse" side. A horse that has systematically been trained will be supple and flexible on both reins.

The lengthways bend is just as important as the sideways bend for the elasticity and suppleness of the gaits. The lengthways bend is only required once the horse has mastered the sideways bending equally on both reins. This mainly consists of the flexion in the haunches and the amount of "give" in the jowls. The term flexion in the haunches is extremely important, and I will allow myself to elaborate a little on that. The term "haunches" includes the hip-, stifle- and hock joints of the horse. With proper flexion of the haunches, these three joints must be equally involved. If the hock is over flexed, one will find early signs of wear, resulting for example in a spavin. Lengthways bending may only be gradually incorporated into the training of the horse, for the muscles and tendons of the horse must first become supple and strong. When gradual gymnastic training is employed, all the above mentioned joints will develop at the same time and acquire a superior degree of elasticity, thrust and weight–bearing capacity. The

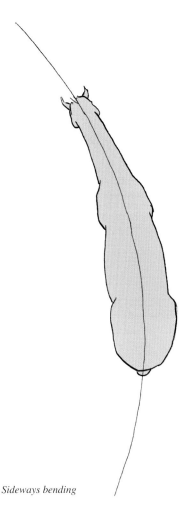

Sideways bending

horse will be supple in all its gaits and as a rule will furthermore be comfortable in its movement under the rider. In achieving this, one of the most important criteria of the art of riding is fulfilled.

Bending, sideways and more specifically lengthways, promotes the improved degree of skill and enhances the suppleness of the horse, thereby also improving balance, contact and collection.

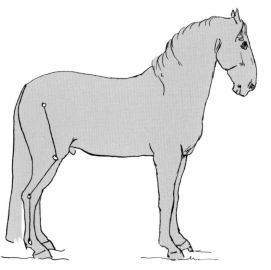

Static bend in the haunches

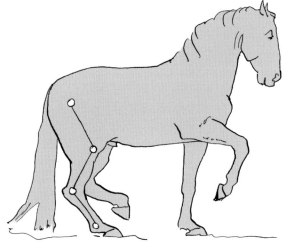

Dynamic bend of the haunches in the piaffe

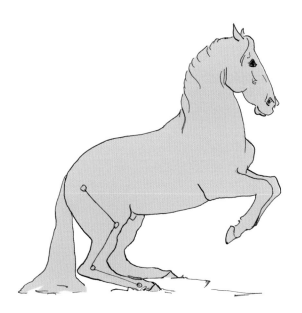

Flexion of the haunches and perfect lengthways bend: the highest possible degree of collection in the levade

The goals of training are always interacting with each other. All the objectives together form the whole, they cannot function on their own or separately from each other.

"In exactly the same manner as the artist will step back to observe the big picture, so must the rider." (Alois Podhajsky, former director of the Spanish Riding School in Vienna.)

Through the correct lengthways bend, a comfortable horse is created for the rider and with that an important requirement of the art of riding is satisfied.

COLLECTION

The term collection is associated with the horse stepping under its body with increased engagement of the hindlegs, and where the centre of gravity of both horse and rider is significant. With energetic forward movement, one can speak of engagement only when the hindfoot overtracks the frontfoot by several centimetres. In collection the hindlegs should already be well engaged under the body of the horse.

Collection is necessary in order to ride the horse in shortened gaits and tight corners and to execute smooth and flowing half-halts. Collection allows a higher degree of flexion of the haunches and thus enables a superior level of athleticism, at the same time preventing early wear on the joints of the horse. Prerequisites for collection are balance, contact and straightness. These objectives also interrelate: in this way collection will enhance the balance and improve the gait as well as the contact. When the horse increasingly steps under its body, it will step even more into the supporting hand of the rider and in doing so will shorten its body.

If the rider can feel the horse stepping under its body on the rein on the same side, it is called "stepping into the rein". Collection will naturally be the result of such a movement. The only time this collection is expected in the halt, is when the rider explains the aids to a young horse or to do a test in the advanced stages of training.

Collection is never accomplished by pulling on the reins or even worse, by using the curb bit. The one and only way of achieving collection is the systematic development of the horse's gymnastic ability and allowing the horse, when it is ready, to step under itself with escalated intensity.

> *As soon as force commences,*
> *art terminates.*

ELEVATION

Elevation is when the head and neck are carried in a much higher position without actually losing the curve in the neck. It is essential for the improvement of balance. Elevation comes about through the mere achievement of collection and may never be forced upon the horse. If the horse is forced into a high head carriage through use of the reins, the result will be a tight back and the loss of balance. This is quite the opposite of what we want to accomplish. The correct elevation is created when the hindquarters lower, producing more flexion in the haunches through the higher degree of collection. The horse gives the illusion of being raised in the front; its movements become more breathtaking, lighter, with added freedom and the hindquarters step under the body with increased impulsion and energy. The hindquarters of the horse act as the engine

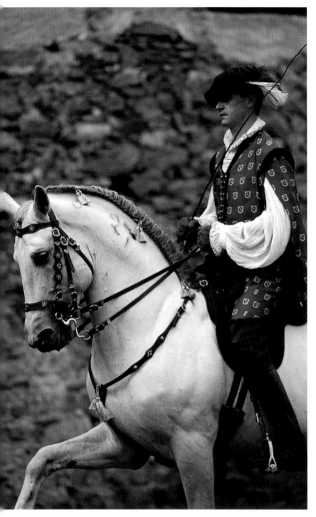

Correct elevation is the result of successful training of a horse

the unbelievable quantities of bits that have been designed all over the world, all to make it easier (?) to achieve the desired elevation. Correct elevation is the result of successful training of the horse, and conformation plays a substantial part here. In horses with weak backs or hindquarters, only a small degree of elevation will be achieved for horses with weak backs tend to hold their heads too high and in the process push their backs away. In such a case the horse in question should first of all be taught to carry the weight of the rider in a swinging fashion in order to strengthen the muscles, but without elevation. The slow process of elevation may be expected only once the hindlegs start to step further under the horse: this is only the beginning. Not every horse will achieve true elevation. It is reserved for those horses whose conformation and characters are suited to high school education. In correct elevation, the crest of the horse's neck will move closer to the rider while the lower part of the neck stays in a concave form. If the lower neck is convex, the neck is "pushed out", a fault that is more often than not caused by too strong a hand from the rider.

> *Elevation is only one of the progressive goals in the art of riding*

and are responsible for the expression of the movements in all the gaits.

The misconceptions surrounding the term "elevation" are as numerous as those that accompany the term „bits". Proof lies in

The different
Techniques of
Working in Hand
and the ways they are employed

Due to the numerous different methods of working the horse in hand, I have endeavoured to divide them into a system. Every style of work in hand can be used completely separately from the others, although with less efficiency. The system that I recommend, training horses using both riding and in hand work, has been shown to be totally effective as well as being kind to the horse.

The system of classical work in hand comprises the following types of groundwork:
· Work on the lunge with or without cavaletti
· Work on the long rein with or without cavaletti
· Classical work in hand according to the Iberian way

· Classical work in hand according to the Viennese way (Spanish Riding School)
· Work in the pillars according to Pluvinel
· Work with shortened long reins.

I would like to give short descriptions of each of these and then continue in more detail on each of them.

WORK ON THE LUNGE

The work that can be done with the lunge rein has the widest variety of possibilities of all the work on the ground. The horse can be exercised, collected, relaxed or simply be moved, all just by utilising the lunge rein.

over cavaletti without a rider. Work on the lunge is regularly criticised, for example the strong influence of centrifugal forces, the physically powerful loading on the joints. The answer to that is simply that horses have been lunged for centuries without any great damage, as long as the work is done in an accomplished manner. As we are all aware, any category of training that is employed incorrectly or used excessively can cause a certain amount of damage. Special attention must therefore be given when working on the suitability of training with young horses, as we are, after all, working with uncoordinated and delicate living creatures. The Spanish Riding School of Vienna is proof that lungeing, correctly implemented, is not at all damaging. Their horses are lunged for two months before they are ridden without a lunge rein attached. Many of the stallions in the Spanish Riding School live to be twenty-six years old and still perform without damage being done before they are pensioned off.

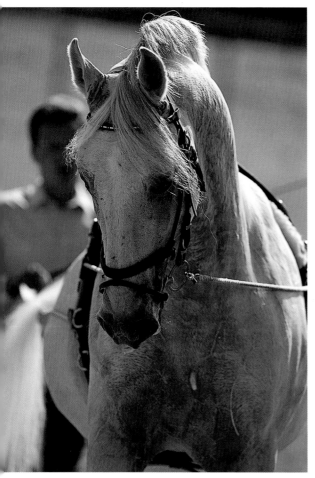

With long reins we can bend, place and teach the horse impulsion

One of the important uses for the lunge is in its employment on the young, unbroken horse. Here you have the possibility of teaching a young horse, without a struggle or bad experience, what is expected from him when training with or without a rider. One will regularly see lungeing used as a warm-up exercise for horses, especially on the Iberian peninsula. Also to be taken into consideration in lungeing is the possibility of working

WORK WITH LONG REINS

Long reining is suitable for every horse that is lunged on a regular basis. It is the natural choice for work on straight lines and for developing impulsion. If the horse is particularly forward going, this is an especially suitable way of training.

With the long reins we can bend and place the horse, and start on the road to impulsion. Long reins are above all recommended for training the horse over poles or cavaletti, but the trainer needs to be superbly dextrous in handling the reins. Collected work is also possible with the long reins, but other ways of work in hand will have preference over this method.

CLASSICAL TRAINING IN HAND ACCORDING TO THE IBERIAN SCHOOL

The work on the Iberian peninsula is quite similar to that of the Viennese school, and is practised there as well. The Iberian manner of work in hand is orientated towards the breeds of horses that live there: for example the Pura Raza Espanol (P.R.E.), also known as the Andalusian, and the Lusitano from Portugal. These horses are extremely spirited and have great manoeuvrability and this is the heart of this work. First of all in this work in hand lateral work is demanded and from there the piaffe, passage and airs above the ground are developed. The Spanish walk and Spanish trot are also requested. The advantage lies in a certain freedom that is allowed the horse, for they are worked without side reins and therefore have a greater opportunity to give and stretch in their contact. The disadvantage lies in the restricted freedom of movement for the trainer, for he must take part in all the move-

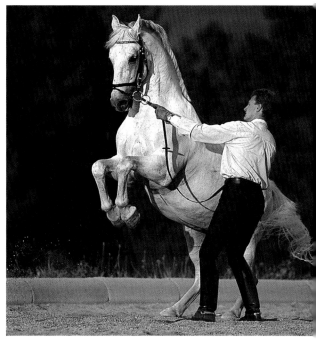

Work in hand according to the Iberian school with the Lippizaner stallion Maestoso Ancona

ments the horse makes and have limited choices where he can use the whip. If you happen to work with an apathetic horse, this type of schooling can be carried out only on a very limited scale, for such a horse will not possess the necessary sensitivity for the vocation. In general, this work is more suited for somewhat responsive horses and can be of real benefit to them. It is also fitting for those horses that have been trained on the ground and have already developed this kind of sensitivity. As a precursor the work on the long reins will be exceedingly useful.

TRAINING IN HAND ACCORDING TO THE VIENNESE SCHOOL

This method of working in hand can most certainly be described as the classical way. It is normally only taught to perfection in the Spanish Riding School of Vienna and has many advantages, but also one or two disadvantages.

One advantage is the ability to obtain the extremely high degree of collection displayed in the gaits of the high school movements, mainly the piaffe and the passage and then the school jumps, the last of which are exclusively trained in this manner. Every single leg and area on the body can be individually and exactly touched with the whip. The biggest disadvantage of this way of working in hand is the lack of impulsion and the loss of forwardness. I only commence with the work in hand according to the Viennese School after the lunge and long rein work have been utilised and then to refine the knowledge and put the finishing touches to the horse.

interested in making use of this technique that they obtain an experienced and knowledgeable trainer, who knows how this technique functions! In the work between the pillars the opportunity arises to perfect and complete the finer points of the piaffe and the airs above the ground.

It is also possible to work around a single pillar, simulating normal lungeing as well as incorporating the lateral exercises. The advantage of work in the pillars is the complete freedom the trainer has to move around the horse whilst facilitating the perfection of the different movements by the horse.

The disadvantage of this kind of work is the fact that the horse can easily get into a forced position from where it will hardly be possible to relax. Work between the pillars can be dangerous work that can cause injury to the horse with incorrect employment.

It is of even more importance that the horse is prepared properly before work between the pillars is attempted.

WORK BETWEEN THE PILLARS ACCORDING TO PLUVINEL

This kind of training is extremely difficult and can be dangerous for the horse when executed in an amateurish fashion. I would like immediately to recommend to anyone

WORK WITH SHORT-ENED LONG REINS

This is considered to be the culmination of work in hand, but it remains only a result of and not a method of training. A horse can only perform in the shortened long reins what it has already learnt under the rider and that training being complemen-

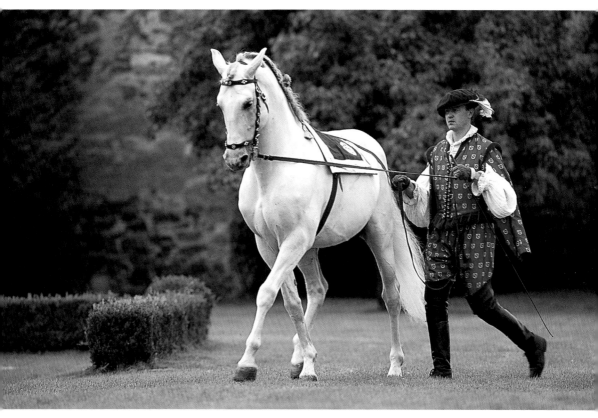

Work on the shortened long reins is the culmination of the work in hand.

ted and perfected by work in long reins. This is where complete expression comes from the horse with only minimal input from the trainer. In order to reach this fulfilment, there are some prerequisites for both horse and rider.

Not only must the rider have an abundance of sensitivity, but also an adequate amount of personal fitness, for the rider must walk behind the horse all the time, even at the canter. Irrespective of the degree of training, the horse can under no circumstances be prone to kicking; it needs to be one hundred per cent trustworthy. A second, not completely unimportant factor is the size of the horse. Horses that are too big have too big gaits to match steps and it is impossible to stay in a walk behind them. Apart from that, very big horses have various other disadvantages of which we shall hear later on in this book.

Work on the Lunge

EQUIPMENT

One of the most important pieces of equipment from the point view of injury to the rider is gloves. If the horse decides to bolt and pulls the rope through the hands of the rider, it can cause significant burns to the hands. Never lunge the horse without gloves!

The next item we need is a lungeing whip that must comply with the following:

· It must not be too heavy; it is used for about a half an hour at a time and sometimes even longer.

· It must be long enough to reach the horse on a circle with a radius of 17-18 metres.

For work in a smaller circle it may be an excellent idea to acquire a shorter lungeing whip as well.

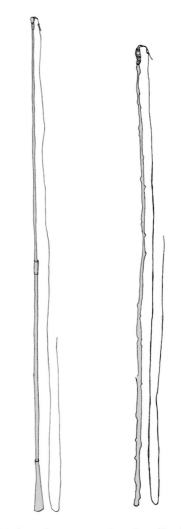

Vaulting whip   *Lungeing whip of natural wood*

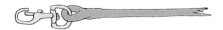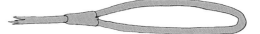

Cotton rope lunge rein as used in the Iberian peninsula

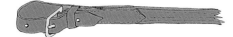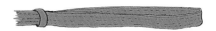

Flat lunge rein, without stoppers, with buckle instead of snap link

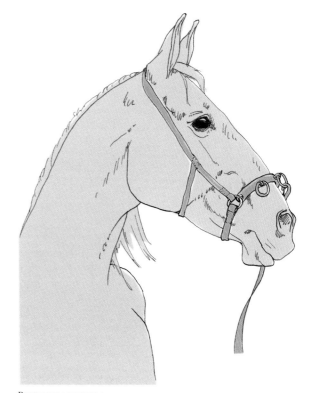

Portuguese cavesson.

Further items of equipment on the list include a lungeing surcingle or roller with an assortment of rings, a headpiece with a snaffle and most importantly in this work, a lungeing cavesson, that has to fit like a glove on the nose of the horse if it is to have any effect on the horse whatsoever. I usually use a cavesson from Spain or Portugal as well as one from the Spanish Riding School; unfortunately the last mentioned is difficult to find. The material from which the lunge rein is made is also extremely important. Among the best is the flat or rolled cotton lunge rein, for cotton is stable and lies well in the hand. It is entirely dependent on your own preference whether you choose a rolled or flat lunge rein. If a rolled rein is preferred, it is advisable that it has some stoppers, whereas this is not necessary on a flat rein. An ideal length for a lunge rein is about 7-8 metres. A lunge of 9-metre length can be utilised on young horses. Further equipment, depending on the type of training, will be side reins or even a chambon. Use of these training aids will be discussed at a later stage.

SKILLS
OF THE TRAINER

An extremely important part of the work on the lunge is the ability of the trainer to use the lunge whip precisely. In the Spanish Riding School it is customary to practise hitting the right target by using empty cans at first. This is an exercise I

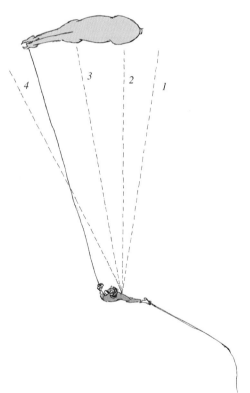

1. *Driving position of the whip.*
2. *Neutral position of the whip:*
   it points to the fetlock, hock or hip joint.
3. *Pushing the horse into a bigger circle.*
4. *Restraining position.*

would recommend to everyone who would like to lunge a horse the correct way. You have to be able to touch the horse at any one point with flick of the whip when the exact moment presents itself. It is easier to start with the whip in the right hand, if you are right-handed. The whip must lie loosely in the hand, the lash pointing to the back; you positively feel the stroke in your hand. Now you tap the lash with a flick of the wrist on a precise target, preferably an empty can. The faster the actual flick is halted or even pulled back, the stronger is the effect it has. This can be in a range from just touching the horse to reprimanding it with the lash.

There are a number of points on the horse that have to be touched according to what is required. This is on the hindleg, in the region between the cannon bone and the point of the buttock, wherever the horse reacts the best to the aid: on this point the whip will have a strong, forward driving message. When the lash is flicked in an upward motion towards the belly, slightly behind the girth, it persuades the horse to jump into a canter. Softly touching the shoulder of the horse will encourage it to move out into a slightly bigger circle. As you can envisage, a great deal of accuracy is required to exclude the possibility of hitting the horse on the head or, worse still, in the eye.

In general, the effect of the whip is punishing when applied in a downward stroke. When used from below or horizontally, it has a more inviting impression. Before actually touching the horse with the whip, one should try other options like the voice or the visual stimulation of the action of the whip first.

The voice plays an important role when working in hand; it can have a calming or stimulating effect, depending on the tone used.

As far as the visual encouragement from the whip goes, that will depend on the trainer and the position where the trainer stands as well as the whip itself. The whip must point to the hock of the horse, in other words the horse must be framed between the lunge rein and the whip. When the suggestion is one of driving the horse forward, the whip is lifted slightly more to the back. When the horse needs to be calmed down or slowed down into the next gait, the whip is held in front of the horse. When the horse closes in on the circle the whip is pointed to the shoulder, if no reaction occurs, the whip can be pointed to the head of the horse. Should the need arise, the trainer can reinforce this visual encouragement by using his position relative to the horse. In this way the horse will react and become more forward moving when the trainer is slightly behind, and will be converted into slower movement when the trainer apparently cuts in front of the horse. Only when all the visual stimuli have been totally ignored by the horse, should the stronger aid of the flick of the whip be administered.

Once you have developed accuracy with both the left and right hands, you can venture to tackle the horse.

Great care must also be given to the technique utilised with the lunge rein. It should not be twisted, but rather be smooth and carefully looped in the hand, taking special caution that the hand cannot be caught in the rein.

TRAINING THE HORSE WITH LUNGEING

There are four reasons to lunge a horse:
· To give it some movement
· To train a rider
· To train the horse
· To correct a horse and release tensions.

I will not go into any depth on the movement of the horse or the training of the rider as these are not the subject matter of this book. I think the section on the seat of the rider (p.18) is more than adequate.

The foundation of work in hand is the lunge work, especially with young, unbroken horses. The objective of this is to win over the trust of the young horse. The horse must learn that it must follow the orders of the rider. The horse must gain balance without the added weight of the rider and learn to become skilled and agile. Once the horse's trust is earned, the road to obedience

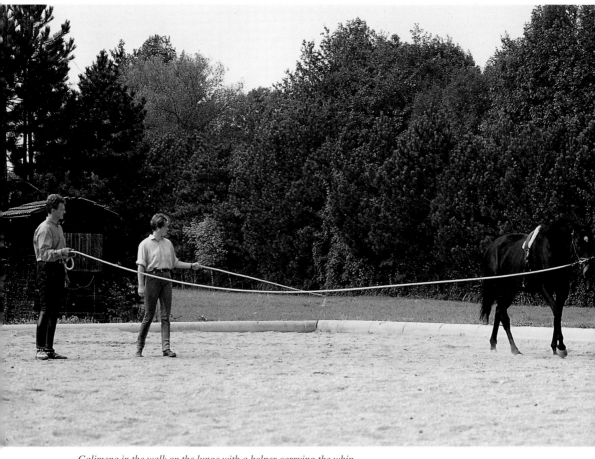

Galimena in the walk on the lunge with a helper carrying the whip

lies open. Another motive for the work on the lunge is for the horse to comprehend the language and aids of the trainer.

Correct lungeing is not an easy task; it is an art in which the horse must move in a circle around the trainer. For a start the horse must get used to the bridle, lungeing cavesson, lungeing roller and saddle most of the time this can be achieved in the stable with a lot of patience. With calm words and slow, definite gestures the horse can quietly become accustomed to the unusual articles we place on it.

At this point we lunge the horse for the first time, dressed in a bridle, cavesson, lungeing roller and side reins. I would like to explain the attachment of the cavesson separately. The horse has a normal snaffle bridle with a soft bit, or a simple head-piece with the bit in will do.

The cavesson is placed over the bridle and the jowl straps buckled in such a way that they lie under the throatlatch of the bridle. The jowl strap must be tight enough for the cavesson not to move towards the eye of the horse when pulled. The noseband of the cavesson must be buckled underneath the bridle to enable the bridle to move freely over the cavesson without injury to the delicate region of the mouth. The reinforced noseband of the lungeing cavesson must lie below the facial crest but above the nasoincisive notch. When the cavesson is in this position the horse can feel the effect without its breathing being interrupted. The choice of cavesson will depend on the sensitivity of the horse's nose. If the horse's nose is exceptionally sensitive, the cavesson must be additionally padded, but no more than those used in the Spanish Riding School, or the effect will be lost completely. The cavesson must not be too tight or too loose, for this will lead to chafe marks on the bridge of the nose. The lunge rein is then attached to the middle ring on the cavesson.

For the first lunge lesson it is recommended to have a helper to man the whip. The helper leads the horse, which has the side reins loosely attached, on the lunge rein in a circle of about 17 metres and slowly moves away from the horse by moving closer to the trainer in the middle of the circle. The side reins are attached so the horse feels the weight of the reins; they must not be adjusted too long or too short, for that will only create resistance. The

correct height for the side reins to be attached to the roller is apparent in the accompanying photographs. Once the horse is ready the trainer can then shorten the side reins in the walk while the helper softly urges the horse to continue if it wants to spontaneously go into a halt. In this manner any possible resistance or panic from the horse can be avoided. With the same careful approach the side reins can also be attached lower on the roller, but they should never be fastened lower than the lowest border of the saddle flap. What the work on the lunge strives for is that the horse gives the impression of searching for contact with the bit in a long and low frame, gently rounding the back in the process. Under no circumstances must the side reins be attached so high that the horse is forced to tighten its back muscles. The conclusive length of the side reins is a matter of the individual and should as a rule of thumb be measured in the fact that the horse does not move with its nose behind the vertical.

In most cases the left side of the horse is considered the easier side and for this reason the horse should be lunged on this side first. The helper holds the whip in the right hand while the trainer holds the lunge rein in the left hand. The middle of the circle is always determined by the inside foot of the trainer, for that is the foot he will move around himself. When the horse follows the helper to the middle of the circle, it must under no circumstances be flicked to the outside with the whip.

In such a situation the helper must calmly lead the horse to the outside of the circle once more until such a time as the horse understands what is expected from him. This leading to the outside of the circle must of course happen at a walk. Once the horse appreciates what is required from him, the whole exercise can be repeated on the other side. On the right side the first difficulties will start to appear. This does not only lie in the fact that the youngster is not very proficient on this rein, but also in the detail that the helper has to carry the whip in the left hand and is not always as skilful in that direction himself. Once the horse moves well in both directions at

a walk, the trot may be attempted on the easy side, with the accompanying request from the trainer's voice and visual stimulation through the lifting of the whip behind the horse. Right from the start the trainer should take tremendous care not to over exert the horse; it is much more sensible if the horse gets used to the exercise slowly. After a few minutes of trot work the horse must be given a breather and walk for one or two minutes before repeating the trot exercise.

The horse must respect, but not fear the whip. The whip must only be used in a gentle manner in the beginning and the preferred aid should be the visual stimulation used with it. If the horse does not react, the lash of the whip can softly be flicked to the area just behind the girth. If this flick touches the horse more to the hindquarters, there is always the likelihood that the young horse will protest by kicking out at it. The whip must never hit the horse anywhere on the head. Apart from the fact that the whip could cause serious injury to the eye, it could also generate acute difficulties with the horse becoming head-shy. The driving feeling of the whip is often enough when the flick is produced behind the horse or when the trainer gives a step towards the horse. When the horse pushes to the middle of the circle while being lunged, the whip handle can be pointed at it – the tip of the whip pointed to the nose or shoulder of the horse. In this way the horse will develop an equal and even contact to the lunge rein and

Trot: when the trainer lifts the lunge rein, the horse moves out to a larger circle

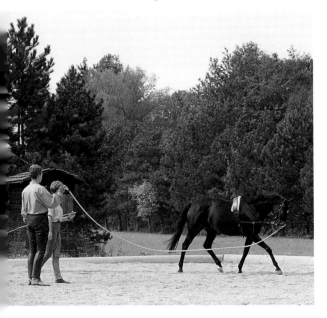

the trainer has more chance to determine the size of the circle and half-halt the horse.

When commencing lungeing with a young horse, it is good practice to select a circle of 17-19 metres in diameter, so the horse can learn to balance easier.

During the work on the lunge the trainer should stand still in one spot and not walk more than the horse, as is often seen. The helper on the other hand, walks closer to the horse just behind the lunge rein. We continue in this manner and shorten the side reins with each lesson until the horse goes in the acceptable bend in the circle.

At this stage it is time to start transitions into halt, walk-trot and even to attempt canter transitions. It is more difficult to execute a complete halt transition with a young horse, for they have a strong yearning to go forward. To begin with the halt is requested from a walk only. The whip is transferred under the lunge rein, or as in vaulting, over the lunge rein, and as a definite visual stimulus held in front of the head. As a voice aid a long stretched out and calm "Whoa" or "Stand" is said. It does not matter what word is used, it depends on the tone applied when saying it. It is important to make use of the same word all the time in order for the horse to react with absolute reliability later on in life. If the horse does not react to these words, the visual stimulus of taking a step toward the horse, almost as if cutting off the way, must be performed. If even that fails to bring the desired result, the half-halt on the cavesson can be employed. The best-proven technique is to shake the lunge rein, for this puts a definite constraint on the bridge of the nose of the horse.

When you want a young horse to canter, it is sensible to use a corner of the arena or better still, a purpose-built lunge ring for this exercise. Before the horse reaches the corner of the arena, I will half-halt the horse once or twice on the cavesson and flick the whip from below, that is from the hock up towards the shoulder. I will simultaneously, as encouragement, say the word "canter" and repeat this until the horse reacts in the desired manner. Once the horse is in control of the canter, I will commence the trot-canter transitions, where the horse trots for a half circle and then canters for a half circle on the lunge until it knows the exact aids for the transitions. The sequence can be shortened according to your wishes, for example three or four canter strides and then a few trot steps, followed by canter again. This exercise can also be done with the walk to trot and trot to walk sequences.

Once the horse is reasonably competent on the lunge, it is time to progress and get onto its back. But do not throw caution to the wind. The first acquaintance with the weight of the rider should be when the rider lies across the saddle on the horse's back. Before this the rider should pat the saddle a couple of times to show the horse there is no need to be frightened if it. The helper gives the rider a leg-up and the rider softly lies over the saddle.

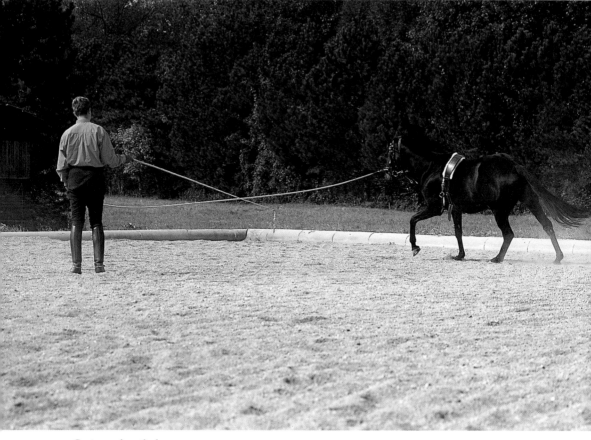

Canter work on the lunge

All of this takes place with an abundance of soothing words and strokes on the neck. Praise is also accepted in the form of titbits – the stomach is the route to to the heart! As soon as the horse does this a few days in a row without being frightened, the trainer can lead the horse a few strides at the walk. The helper must hold onto the legs of the rider when the horse walks to prevent the rider from falling head over heels over the other side. As soon as the horse appears to be competent, the whole exercise is repeated with the rider sitting upright in the saddle. Here again the rider should be given a leg-up by the helper. When the horse is accustomed to the weight of the upright rider, the lessons on the lunge must recommence in the same order as without any rider. The basic gaits of the horse are now performed until the horse's balance is established.

The transition and halts are only brought into play at a later stage; the same goes for the rein back, until the horse is confident in performing them. In the meantime the horse must be lunged without the aid of a helper.

Now is the time to ride the horse without the assistance of the lunge rein. At the onset of the lesson it is wise to lunge the horse to warm it up without the extra weight of the rider, and to achieve the so-called "working temperature". In the first lesson off the lunge, the helper leads the horse on a lead rein attached to the cavesson, with an older experienced horse in front of the young horse to keep things as unproblematic as possible. I would personally ride all the young horses with the help of the cavesson combined with the snaffle bit, for the simple reason that the horse already knows the effect of the cavesson. A second set of reins is attached to the rings on the nosepiece of the cavesson – the horse is then ridden with two sets of reins. Starting the horse in this way has the advantage that the horse's mouth can stay delicate. Gradually the horse can then be ridden on the snaffle rein only and the cavesson can be completely abandoned.

The lesson in the arena can become more demanding with the inclusion of straight lines as well as riding in circles. As this progresses the young horse will frequently develop problems with going in straight lines, and start to stagger. This stems from the fact that the horse has learnt to balance itself on a circle on the lunge and needs to develop this capability on straight lines as well. During the work on the lunge with the rider, the side reins must be attached in a much longer frame and the rider must endeavour to get the horse between hand and leg. The connection between the horse's mouth and the rider's hand must always be very elastic. The rider must attempt to present an enjoyable sensation in the horse's mouth in order to stimulate the chewing on the bit. This can only be done with the help of the correct forward driving aids. The influence may never come from a left and right sawing motion on the reins, for this will teach the young horse to swing its head from side to side to keep in rhythm. When the lunge circle is made smaller with or without the rider, it can help the horse to find its balance in tighter turns. The important thing is not to exaggerate this and teach the horse to swing out its hindquarters on the circle.

In the warming up phase the downward transitions are extremely important, from trot to walk, canter to trot and the halt. As soon as the horse is somewhat warmed up, the distances between the transitions can be shortened and the horse needs to be quicker at the changes, as a result training the body and the mind of the horse at the same time. Within a short space of time you will notice that the horse starts to think quicker and will become bored by too many repetitions very easily. You can ask your horse to think and should never punish the horse's own inventiveness, especially if it goes in the right direction.

If your horse offers something voluntarily it is an excellent sign, for this means he is enjoying himself and that is what we have in mind! When the horse volunteers something at the beginning it should actually be praised to increase the enjoyment he has at actually learning something new. At a later stage, however, the horse should not be praised but ignored, for the lesson must be instigated at the request of the rider. If these little sessions from the horse become too regular, it is advisable to divert the horse's attention by doing something else and to encourage the horse to obey the rider more. If the time and place of the aids are varied, it teaches the horse to wait for the aids from the rider.

A further aspect of the work on the lunge will now come into play, namely the work with cavaletti.

LUNGEING OVER CAVALETTI

The main goal of training a riding horse, regardless of it being a jumper or a dressage horse, is gymnastic exercise. The muscles grow stronger and the joints and tendons more supple. In the work over the cavaletti, the horse is encouraged to control its movements and at the same time develop more energy and stride with more elevation over the obstacle. An additional benefit of work over cavaletti is that it is just the thing to loosen the muscles and prevent the onset of tightness. Horses that are regularly worked over cavaletti will furthermore develop a higher degree of surefootedness and will also learn to quickly and efficiently lower their centre of gravity. The use of cavaletti will make the training of a young horse effortless and add variety to the daily chores!

Apart from the normal lungeing gear, the extra equipment will come in the form of cavaletti. It is not recommended to use plain poles on the ground, for the chance of injury when the poles roll away is excessively high. It is especially necessary to protect the legs of the horse when working over cavaletti and therefore it should normally wear bandages or protective boots.

The different gaits will require the cavaletti to be placed different distances apart. Walk: approximately 80 centimetres apart, trot: approximately 120 centimetres apart, canter: approximately 300 centimetres apart. These, however, are only guidelines, the stride-length of the individual horse will determine the distance between the cavaletti.

When working on the lunge, the cavaletti have to be spaced at regular intervals for the work is performed on a circle. Another option is to put the cavaletti on every quarter of the circle. This will allow for more freedom in the gaits; the horse can perform all gaits without changing the distances between the cavaletti. If the trainer can move along the long side of the arena with the horse, the cavaletti can be

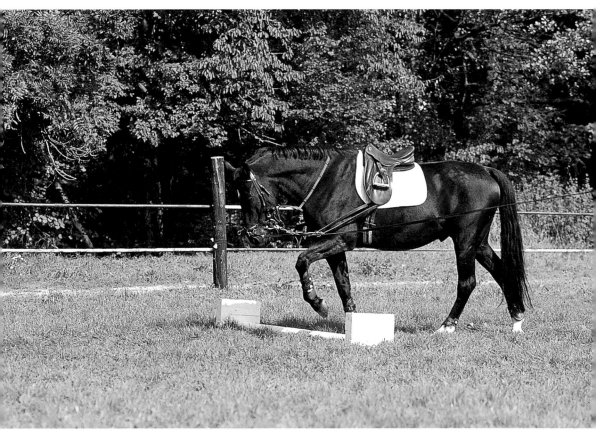

Don Pedro working over cavaletti at the walk

spaced on a straight line along the arena. When this method is used the horse already has to be experienced in the work on the lunge.

Cavaletti work at the trot

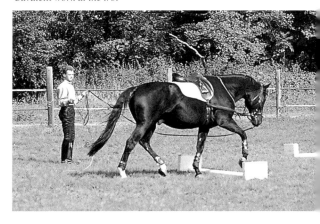

It is extremely important to issue a warning: take great care when working over cavaletti, the lunge can easily catch on the side of the cavaletti with very unpleasant results.

It is more appropriate to let the horse get accustomed to the work over the cavaletti at a slow pace, for this work is not without risk. Horses that are not familiar with this

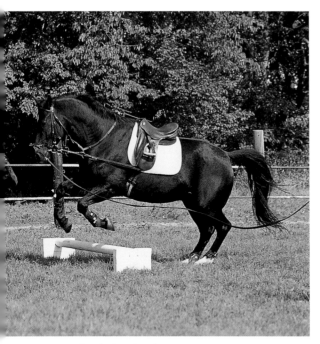

Cavaletti work at the canter

Work in the trot over several cavaletti

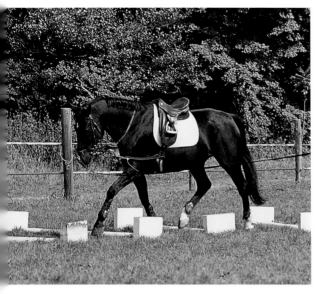

procedure will tend to stumble if there are too many cavaletti at once, resulting in the possibility of falls and associated lameness. Remember - less is more in this situation! At the beginning only one or two cavaletti should be placed in the circle for the horse.

Once the trainer is satisfied that the horse can successfully step over more than one at a time, others can be added. In the work on the lunge, the quantity of cavaletti is limited because the work is executed on a circle.

Cavaletti work is started off at the walk and then upgraded to the trot. These two gaits can be greatly enhanced with the work over the cavaletti. Canter work over cavaletti has always been a matter for discussion, for many trainers suggest this can only productively be utilised when the horse is trained for show jumping and the surefootedness and rhythm of the horse needs to be improved upon. Gymnastic exercises from a dressage point of view means that the elasticity, rhythm and push from the hindquarters will be developed to a higher standard. These horses become more skilled with the placement of their legs, which shows up across country, and learn to use their backs by stepping right under their bodies in soft bouncy movements.

At the same time as starting the work over cavaletti without the rider on the lunge, the training of the horse over cavaletti with the rider on board both on and off the lunge must commence. The work on the lunge should now be gradually

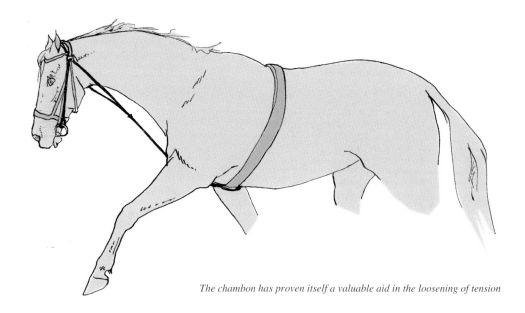

The chambon has proven itself a valuable aid in the loosening of tension

reduced to not more than twice a week. This work should also be without the help of the side reins with just the possibility of a martingale attached as aid. Work over the cavaletti should not be performed more than twice a week and must rather be a welcome substitute in the daily routine of the horse.

LOOSENING TENSION THROUGH LUNGEING

The next purpose for which the work on the lunge can be utilised with great success is to loosen the tension in a horse with a tight back. There are two pieces of equipment that have proved to be valuable in this task and they are the equilunge and

the chambon. The biggest advantage the equilunge has over the chambon lies in the fact that I have never met a horse that has resisted this method whereas it can sometimes happen with the chambon. Both of the pieces of equipment named above have proven to be ideal in the work over cavaletti as well, allowing for the forward and down stretch and not the high head carriage that accompanies a tightened back.

The application of this equipment must be unhurried and the horse must gradually be accustomed to its use. The length must be shortened little by little until the horse has the desired outline. Once that is achieved, the work on the lunge can be performed as mentioned previously.

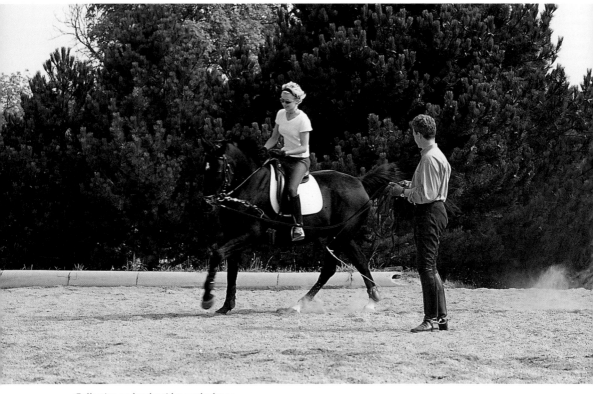

Collection under the rider on the lunge

COLLECTION ON THE LUNGE

Up until now the work on the lunge has been about relaxing the horse in a lengthened stretch at work, but now it becomes progressively obvious that the horse should start to work in a more collected frame.

When is the horse ready to be collected without overtaxing it? As soon as the horse can manage the lessons of rein back, canter-trot transitions, halt from the trot, the impulsion stimulating exercises like medium trot and medium canter as well as shoulder in (see Lateral work p. 72) on the lunge and under the rider, this indicates the point in time when collection can be attempted. Collection on the lunge is recognised purely in the size of the circle used, around 13 metres diameter that can additionally be reduced to 7 metres.

For the time being, first the sequence of events in a lesson that includes collection on the lunge:

The horse is equipped in identical manner as for the customary work on the lunge. Bandages or brushing boots can be added for extra protection. The horse does not wear the side reins tight yet and diligently moves on the normal lunge circle. Once the horse is properly warmed up, the side reins are attached, not too short at the beginning, but high enough up the roller to request some elevation without placing the horse in an artificial posture.

The side reins are attached in such a manner that they incline towards the horizontal when the horse is properly tacked up. At first the horse works on a large circle. Once the horse is visibly relaxed, the actual work of collection can commence.

The horse now is attached on a shorter side rein and the diameter of the lunge circle is reduced to some extent, depending on the capability if the horse, which you will recognise by whether or not the horse throws his haunches out of the circle. Subject to how the horse reacts, the circle can then be reduced or increased. The first training goals of the smaller circle are full halts from the walk, the trot-walk and canter-trot transitions with ever increasing collection. The work on this is maintained until the horse is capable of cantering in a collected manner on a 7-metre circle. It is, however, important to remember that horses, like humans, cannot maintain high performances without some form of relaxation. The horse must then every now and then canter in a larger circle in a more relaxed way, to prevent tension deverloping from toning.

The next step is for the horse to be collected under the rider, who can frame the horse in an even more collected way.

Once this stage of training is reached with the help of the classical work on the lunge, it is time to resume the work on the long reins.

Training format on the lunge

· Getting used to the equipment,
  for example saddle and bridle
· Lungeing the young horse
· Careful riding of the young horse
· Combined lunge and ridden work,
  work on straight lines
· Lunge and ridden work over cavaletti,
  improving rhythm and impulsion
· Reducing the diameter of the circle
  on the lunge and under the rider
  to improve the weight-bearing ability
· Start of the work on long reins.

Work
with
Long Reins

Following on from the work on the lunge, work on the long reins offers countless more possibilities. It is the next step in the complete and systematic training of the horse in hand recommended in this book. Now the trainer can improve the bend, elevation and different school figures and work on the numerous gaits of high school movements.

EQUIPMENT

We need the following equipment for the work with long reins:

· A cavesson for the young horse as in the lunge work. It is, however, important that the cavesson has three rings. Later a bridle with a snaffle bit or a simple D-ring curb bit can be utilised to refine the training.

· A roller with four rings and two 14-metre long cotton long reins, 3 centimetres wide. The reins must have snap hooks on the end running into 2 metres of rolled cotton, which then tapers onto the flat part of the reins.

· Lungeing whip, driving whip and long dressage whip.

Work with the long reins is always started with the reins attached to the cavesson and not the bit of the bridle. This is done in order not to punish the horse's mouth unduly and the aids are in principle the same as on the lunge.

If the trainer works directly behind the horse, as is the case with the advanced work, the dressage whip or the driving whip is used.

The long rein is attached through the third ring of the cavesson and threaded through and attached to the rings of the roller; the outside long rein is passed over the back through the ring in the roller and tied to the last ring on the cavesson. In this way I achieve the normal lead over the nose, especially when working with a young horse that does not know the use of the second rein and this allows the horse to get accustomed to the strange feeling of a rein on the other side of the body. The outside rein regulates the tempo with half-halts and increases the diameter of the circle and, apart from that, has no other function for the time being. The trainer now works in much the same way as on the lunge in the transitions of all three gaits. Once the horse is comfortable with this, the trainer will carefully place the outside long rein over the croup to go around the hindquarters. The effect of the rein on the outside of the hindquarters must be exceptionally sensitive, for the protraction and retraction of the hindleg will cause the rein to shorten and lengthen in an irregular way if the hand does not complement the movement. As soon as the horse is familiarised with the rein around the hindquarters, which is supposed to prevent the hindquarters from falling out, the inside long rein is threaded through the ring on the roller and then attached to the last ring on the cavesson. From this point in time the trainer has the opportunity to use almost all school figures in any way his skill and fitness allows.

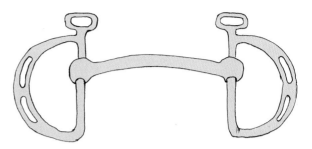

The straight Kimblewick combines the advantages of the snaffle with the minimal leverage of a curb bit: extremely well suited for work with long reins

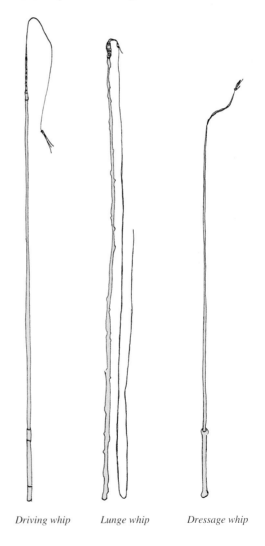

Driving whip   *Lunge whip*   *Dressage whip*

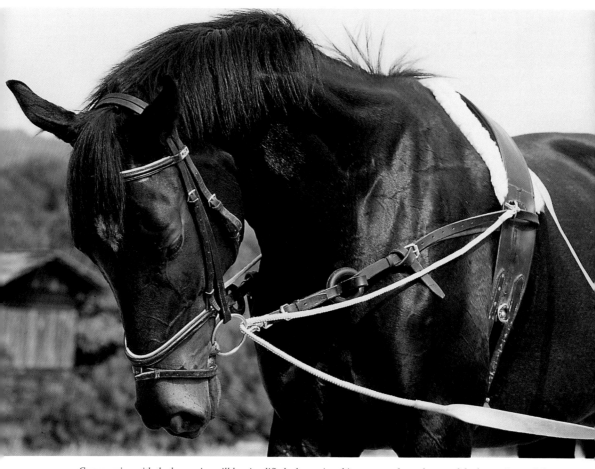

Commencing with the long reins will be simplified when using this manner of attachment of the long reins and the side reins

Allow me a few words about skill and fitness: dealing with the long reins and the whip at the same time will more than likely throw you into the depths of despair at first! Do not lose heart, but cheerfully continue practising until you get the knack of it! The fitness needed to walk behind the horse for a prolonged time will soon come. Remember to pay attention to the ends of

the reins; ensure that the lines lie in ordered and medium length loops in your hand. When the loops are too short, the trainer will have too much rope in the hand and when they are too long, there is a definite danger of tripping on them.

If the trainer uses only one hand for both long reins, the forefinger separates the two lines. The acid test will be when

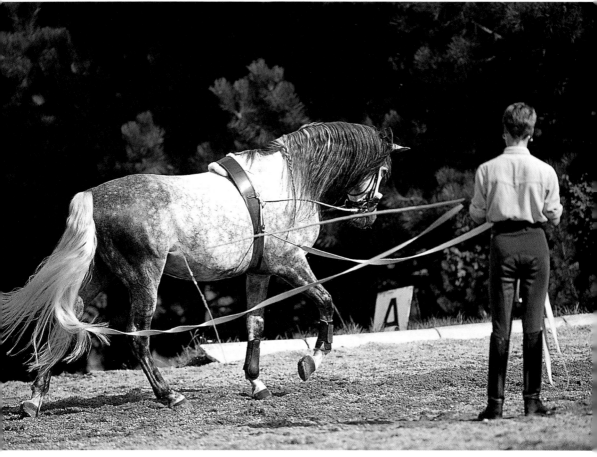

Work at the walk on the circle: even if the long rein ends are of rope, it does not prevent them twisting

the change of rein is demanded. The trainer must then shorten the new inside rein by about 1.5 metres and lengthen the new outside rein by a similar amount at the same time. The whip must be held under the armpit while the change of rein takes place so that it does not become entangled. The change of rein normally takes place on the circle with the horse performing an "s-bend", but can also be performed in a lesson as a volte, off the track.

As soon as the horse performs the transitions and changes of rein with self-confidence, the cavesson is substituted with the normal working bridle the rider will use.

When you first work on the bridle I would like to recommend you use a snaffle with a gag connection to the cheek piece of

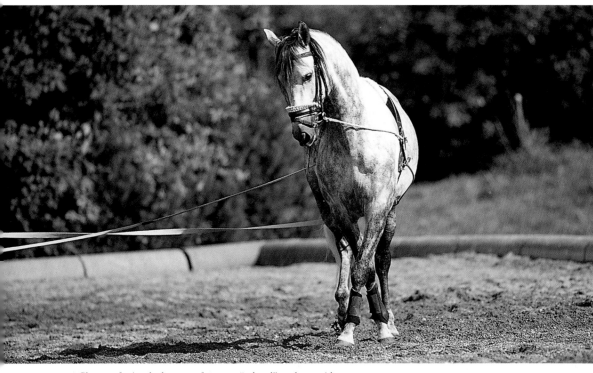

Change of rein: the horse performs an "s-bend" to the outside

Threading the rein through the pulleys
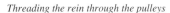

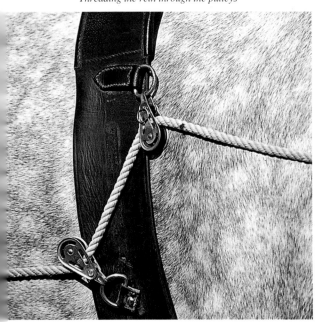

the bridle. The long reins should now also be attached through the rings or pulleys on the roller to formulate a design that goes directly to the mouth of the horse. The smaller the amount of friction the better; excellent pulleys can be bought from good specialist stores for yachting gear.

Another tip for the long reins: you can find rope and reins for all tastes. Do not be scared to experiment to find the material that best suits your needs.

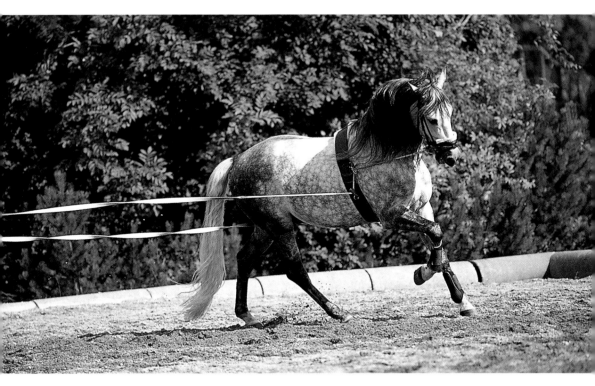

Canter on the circle

GYMNASTIC SCHOOL FIGURES

When the horse is accustomed to the basic rules of long reining, the trainer can run through all the school figures he can think of, first in walk and later in trot. There are countless school figures and some of these have particular gymnastic qualities.

One that especially stands out is the volte or small turn. The volte has the same effect on the well-trained horse that the normal circle has on the young horse that is ridden for the first time. When correctly executed on the long reins or under the rider, it tests the horse's suppleness, balance and agility. Many riders are, despite a fair amount of experience, not capable of riding a correct, round volte.

The volte was originally described as a circle with a 6-metre diameter, while the small turn can be a circle of up to 10 metres in diameter. Both the volte and the small turn are round and neither angular nor elliptic in shape. The volte is an important figure to train a young horse with. In order to make it easier for the horse, the first volte is performed starting

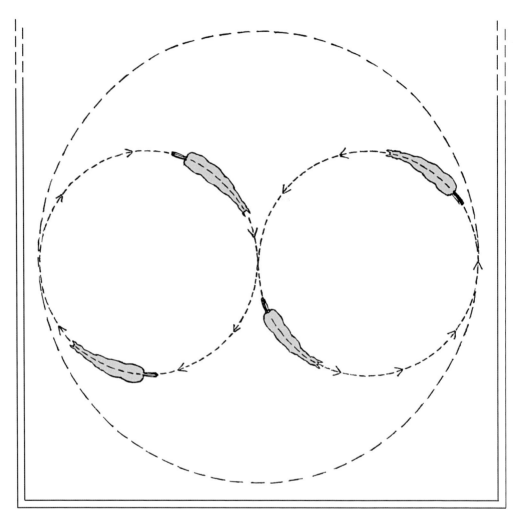

The figure eight within the circle

in the corner of the arena, where the border of the arena outlines two sides of the half circle. The inside rein is shortened and the trainer stays in the middle of the circle of the volte or walks on a small circle himself.

The outside rein, the one around the croup of the horse, forms a border around the horse and prevents the croup from falling to the outside. The volte is divided onto four parts; four quarter turns to be exact. On every quarter the trainer must give the horse a half-halt with the outside rein without losing the bend or contact in the process. To drive the horse forward, the trainer must make use of a driving whip.

When the horse is ridden the rider will show the horse the way with the inside rein. The inside leg of the rider must demand the appropriate bend to the inside, and lies on the girth. At the same time the inside leg ensures that the rhythm and flow of the movement stays the same, while the outside leg is positioned behind the girth to prevent the hindquarters from falling out, and to support the bend from the inside leg. The outside rein determines the size of the volte and the angle of the head. Both seat bones are loaded with identical weight; the rider must never collapse to the inside of the circle or plunge to the outside with his weight. When the rider sits with his weight in the opposite direction to the movement, the horse will stray from the line of the volte, for the horse will undoubtedly follow the weight of the rider.

Impulsion and rhythm must never be lost, whether the horse is on the long rein or under the rider. As part of the preparation for the volte, the normal circle can be reduced until it is around 8-10 metres in diameter. The horse must not travel more than three circuits of this small circle, to avoid the danger of overtaxing it. Afterwards the volte can be ridden at any position in the arena, both on the track and on a free trail in the school. In the latter situation the trainer must remember that the volte is closed: that means it ends where it began.

The school figure that naturally follows out of the volte is the change of rein within the circle in a figure of eight. The most important ingredient in this school figure is precision with the long reins. This lesson increasingly improves the suppleness of the horse with regards to the amount of sideways bend and the elevation. When long reining, the trainer can often get into a spot of trouble with the two reins – shortening and lengthening them takes some practice. In the change of rein the new outside rein is lengthened somewhat while the new inside rein needs to be shortened to some extent. The equivalent aids as described for the volte are valid under the rider. In the change of the rein the horse is first straightened before the new bend is requested. To prevent the horse lifting its head, the light opposite resistance of the new outside rein therefore accompanies change of rein. Frequent changes in the gait, halts and different sized circles used in the eight will lead to more attentiveness from the horse. A separate point to keep in mind is that the horse does not lean to the inside of the half circle with its weight or even fall in with its shoulder. Containing this can be achieved with the help of the outside rein and the inside leg aid, or on the long reins the outside rein and whip that points to the shoulder or neck.

Circles as tight as those just described must in the beginning be attempted only in walk and trot. Canter on the long rein is not expected until a good deal later, when the horse is capable of such elevated and collected canter strides that the trainer can keep up with the horse in a walk. The can-

ter under the rider is performed and established parallel to the other gaits.

LATERAL WORK

The subject matter of lateral work includes all
the movements where the horse not only
moves forward but also sideways. These lateral
gaits may only be expected after analogous
gymnastic training over a sufficient amount of
time.

The old masters always believed that these
are the most difficult lessons for a horse, for
they truly have to be taught to the horse,
regardless of whether from the ground or
mounted. Even horses that are natural masters
of lateral work have to be encouraged to execute these movements correctly or they will
only carry them out in an unsatisfactory manner. Lateral work has an amazing amount of
gymnastic value for the horse, for it demands
freedom of the shoulders, elevation, suppleness
and bend, all of them foundations of the art of
riding.

The following lateral movements have been
known for centuries:

· Leg-yielding
· Shoulder in
· Renvers
· Haunches in
· Travers
· Half pass

LEG-YIELD

The first lesson our horse must learn is the
leg-yield. This exercise should not be given
more substance than necessary. It is not used
for more than the original purpose in the
Spanish Riding School, this being for the
horse to comprehend the sideways driving
aid of the rider's leg. Uninformed use of the
leg-yield and especially its over-use will be
detrimental to the horse. This exercise is
requested from the horse in walk at first or
even in the halt. At the halt it is only asked
under the rider and in the following way:
when the horse halts, and is standing with
its weight evenly on all four legs, the rider
takes his leg slightly behind the girth and
squeezes the leg against the side of the horse,
expecting it to move away from the pressure,
while the rein on the same side supports it.
The reaction of the horse is to step away
from the pressure by crossing its legs when
it moves away. As soon as the first reaction is
made, the horse must be praised and the
exercise must be repeated.

The Iberian way is an especially good
technique to use for the first lesson in leg-
yielding. This exercise can then be continued into a full turn on the forehand. In classical dressage the turn on the forehand is
only a way to a goal, while the way of Doma
Vaquera on the Iberian peninsula utilises
this as a specialised lesson for working with
young bulls. Once the horse accepts the sideways push of the driving leg, the leg-yield is
carried out in the walk and trot as well. The
long rein can additionally be employed in

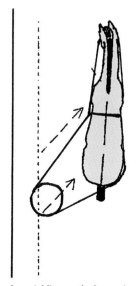

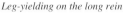

Leg-yielding on the long rein

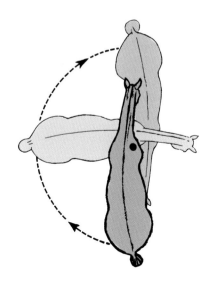

Turn on the forehand

this lesson. The most straightforward way to perform the leg-yield in the long reins is to start from the midline. The driving whip adopts the function of the sideways push of the leg when leg-yielding is done in the long reins.

SHOULDER IN

The first authentic and exceedingly important lesson in lateral work that every horse must learn is the shoulder in. Guérinière was the first master to realise its gymnastic significance, and he elaborated on this topic in his book "Ecole de Cavalerie". In the shoulder in the horse is bent around the inside leg and in the forehand, both shoulders are moved approximately one stride to the inside of the track. The actual

direction of movement is in the opposite direction to that in which the head is pointing. The outside feet step in front of the inside feet. Much greater flexion is demanded from the hock of the inside hindleg in the shoulder in and as the shoulders develop more freedom in their movement, this demand for flexion is increased.

There are two fundamental approaches in the performance of the shoulder in: the shoulder in on three tracks that is expected from horses in competition, and the shoulder in on four tracks, that is mainly presented in the classical manner on Baroque-type horses like the Spanish and Portuguese horses. In order to see the difference between the shoulder in ridden on three tracks and on four tracks, one

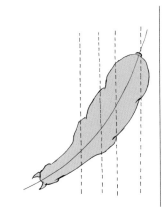

Shoulder in on four tracks

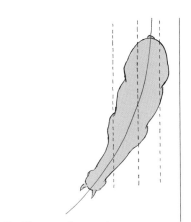

Shoulder in on three tracks

should look from the front; if three legs are visible, it is the shoulder in on three tracks, for the inside hindleg is hidden by the outside front leg as they move on the same track. Shoulder in on four tracks is obviously when all four legs of the horse are visible, for it indicates greater bend in their bodies. The latter is the way that Guériniére discovered and is used to this day in the classical riding institutes and on the Iberian peninsula. According to Guériniére, the Spanish Riding School of Vienna, and myself, the purpose and meaning of the shoulder in is only complete in the version on four tracks. The function and value is namely: the flexion of the hocks, the shoulder becomes free, the contact lighter and the skill and suppleness of the horse is increased.

When the lesser bend is requested in the shoulder in, it can too easily be converted into a leg-yield and in the leg-yield there is no requirement for flexion in the hocks! As is the case in the lesser shoulder in, the shoulder in with too much bend is meaningless. The correct amount of bend in the shoulder in is as important as the fact that it must be performed in identical fashion on both reins. If the horse is ridden on four tracks on the one rein and on less than four tracks on the other rein, the exercise loses its gymnastic usefulness and the horse does not benefit from the training.

All horses have one side, usually the right side, on which they find it easier to execute the bend required from them. This follows on from the fact that they can effortlessly accept the connection with the bit on the one rein and not on the more difficult side, which is usually the left side. All lateral work and the opposing exercises on the long rein will complement the ridden work. I teach the horse the lateral gaits like the shoulder in and renvers, on the long reins as well as under saddle, from the trot. The trot has more impulsion than the walk and is naturally an advantage for this type of work. The most stress-free way to teach a horse the shoulder in, both under the rider and in hand, is out of a circle. The prerequisite is a lively, already shortened trot, even contact on the reins and the horse on the correct bend in the circle. On the long rein the trainer must move the inside shoulder of the horse a little more towards the inside of the circle while the outside rein prevents just the neck from bending. The inside rein is further responsible for maintaining the bend to the inside and the outside rein is responsible for the amount of contact. The long whip is then held on the inside of the horse's body at the exact position where the leg of the rider would be and maintains the bend in the horse's body in this way. The sideways bend must be equal from the head to the tail of the horse. The outside rein around the hindquarters of the horse will at the same time prevent the quarters from falling out.

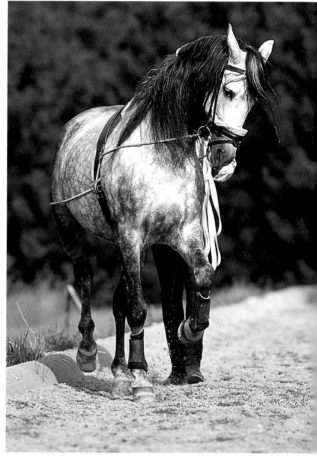

Shoulder in at trot: the horse is attentive, has good contact and bend

Under the rider the aids will be identical, the only difference being the presence of the rider's legs. The rider's inside leg, with the knee held deep, is held against the horse on the girth to encourage the bend in the body and the stepping under of the horse's inside hindleg and the stepping over of the inside foreleg. The outside leg lies slightly behind the girth and prevents the hindquarters from falling out while at the same time maintaining the forward drive.

The supple seat, adapted to the sideways bend of the horse, moving the body weight of the rider in the direction of the shoulder in without restraint, will maintain the impulse of the collected movement of the shoulder in. In the beginning

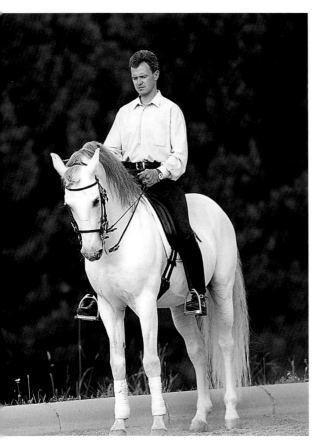

Always correct: halt from the shoulder in

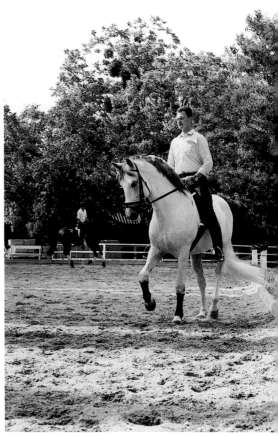

*The author on the Lusitano stallion Cartucho:
shoulder in on the right rein*

the horse is expected to perform only a few steps of shoulder in and then is asked to continue on a circle again. This prevents over taxation and the loss of impulsion of the horse. Once the horse is confident in the shoulder in, the trainer asks for it to be performed from a volte along the long side of the arena.

COUNTER SHOULDER IN

When the counter shoulder in needs to be performed from the straight line, the trainer must place the horse in the opposite bend with opposite contact and direct the horse to the second track after the corner of the arena in order to lead the shoulder of the horse to the outside.

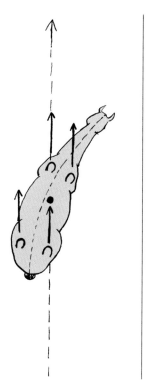

The aids for the counter shoulder in are the exact opposite to those of shoulder in.

FAULTS IN THE SHOULDER IN, AND HOW TO RESOLVE THEM

Counter lessons are almost always exceptional ways to correct faults.

One of the faults that can occur in the shoulder in is the crooked head carriage that is recognisable by the fact that one ear is carried lower than the other. The fault nearly always originates from a really tight outside rein where the horse turns the poll and resists the correct contact on the rein. The horse will generally have a lower inside ear and this can usually be rectified by lifting the inside hand somewhat. If this mistake develops on the long reins and does not resolve when the outside rein becomes more giving and elastic, it is normally a sign that the horse is not yet ready for the shoulder in. In this instance it is better to go back one step and work on the bend on curved lines until the horse becomes more flexible and accepts a better contact.

Loss of impulsion and contact on the long reins:

This fault is easiest corrected if the shoulder in is often changed on the diagonals or more variety is put in such as working on the second track and later on the midline.

Running away and leaving the track:

In this instance I would recommend the shoulder in at the trot to be half-halted into a shoulder in at the walk and to trot again without loss of bend, contact or position.

It is important to have definite constraining inside aids (the whip on the inside girth or inside leg in the ridden work) as the support of the border of the arena is not there. In general, the aids for the counter shoulder in are exactly the same as for the normal shoulder in, but in reverse. In this exercise the trainer should pay extra attention that the horse does not attempt to do a leg-yield instead of the counter shoulder in. This will avoid the meaning of the exercise, which is better contact and bend.

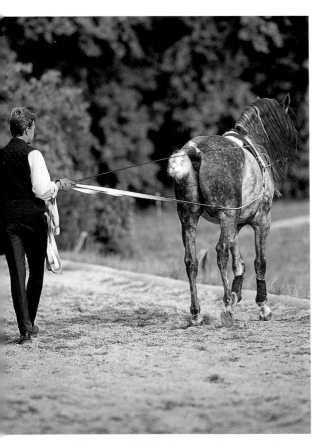

The counter shoulder in: counter lessons are often excellent ways to correct faults

Later, once the horse can master this exercise without difficulty, the trainer can ask the horse to perform a halt in the shoulder in and then trot out of this halt again. Walk-trot transitions are also viable for this situation, although they do not have the same gymnastic effects. The counter shoulder in is the lesson I would recommend to rectify this fault.

Insufficient use of the inside hindleg:
This fault eliminates the whole point of the gymnastic effect – the horse does not step under its body and because of that, there is no flexion in the hocks. Added drive to the hindleg, using the whip on the outside to create more impulsion will help to rectify this fault. The problem almost always comes from the rider or trainer pulling the horse's head in too much, while this at the same time causes the loss of impulsion.

Loss of rhythm:
See loss of impulsion.

Excessive bend in the horse's body:
In this situation the best solution is to make use of the counter shoulder in. This is the best way to correct the wrong bend in the horse's body. Straight after that the horse is positioned in shoulder in. If the horse proceeds in an excessive bend, the trainer must immediately bend the horse in the opposite direction; once that is done, the horse is straightened and then asked for the shoulder in once more with the correct amount of bend. This is repeated a few times until the horse stays in the correct bend.

RENVERS
According to modern opinion, the renvers is achieved in the following way: counter bend – position the horse with the shoulders on the second track while the hindquarters stay on the outside track – bend and contact in the direction of move-

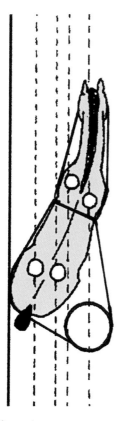

Renvers on long reins

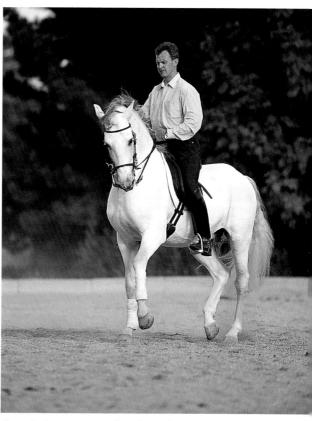

Cartucho in renvers away from the track

ment. The renvers is a difficult lesson, but in a different way from the shoulder in.

Guériniere called this the "croupe au mur", croup to the wall. The horse must move on four tracks. Renvers on the left rein means the trainer must walk on the left side of the horse; on the right rein the trainer walks on the right side. It is superfluous to say that the renvers is to be done in sitting trot. In the Spanish Riding School of Vienna there is classical manner of obtaining the performance of the renvers: shoulder in – from the shoulder in passade, a turn on the haunches in trot (the horse will be approximately 3-5 metres away from the track), from this the transition is made into the half pass and on the track the transition is made into renvers. In the Spanish Riding School this is called shoulder in-passade-renvers in the shortened version. The significance of this is to give rise to a more supple horse in the lateral work and to expect an immediate reaction from the legs.

What is more, the renvers is also an excellent counter lesson for the shoulder in!

TRAVERS AND HALF PASS

Half pass is in principle the identical lesson as the travers; the only difference is that it is not performed on the track of the arena. The travers, which is presented on the track, has a few drawbacks, and for these reasons it is rarely performed in the Spanish Riding School: the majority of horses are prone to be crooked in any case and this lesson will only reinforce this disposition.

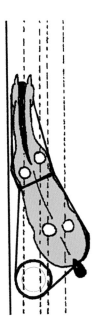

Travers
on long reins

The use of the travers should therefore be reserved for special and exceptional events only. The crookedness of the horse must never be mistaken for a travers with little bend. The intended goal is a bend of the hindquarters, the increasing of the bend and to gain obedience to the leg of the rider. It can be utilised where horses tend to tighten the one side of their bodies and then move crookedly. It can be employed in the following manner: if the horse is stiff on the left rein for example, and moves with the croup slightly towards the inside of the arena, I will do shoulder in on the left rein and travers on the right hand, this is one of the few places where travers has proven itself. The travers is also suited to correcting a horse that reacts in a clumsy and lethargic manner to the leg aids. Here it is best to switch between shoulder in and travers frequently, even more than once on the long side. This will cause more obedience to the leg aids and the horse's skilfulness will be improved. As already described in the shoulder in, the travers can be attempted from the volte as well. Travers should, however, not be given more attention than has been already shown.

The development of the lesson of half pass should also be commenced on long reins and under the rider at the same time. The seat and the influence of the rider here have an extremely important function. The inside rein ensures the appropriate contact without forcing it, the inside leg keeps the forward impulsion.

The outside leg, slightly behind the girth, and supported by the outside hand, encourages the horse to step sideways. The weight of the rider has a natural slant in the direction of the movement, the inside stirrup has more weight in it, and the rider looks in the direction he is moving.

The aids on the long reins: the trainer steps sideways into the middle of the arena, the inside rein bends the horse and leads it into the half pass, with the low outside rein the trainer takes the croup into the half pass and prevents the hindquarters from falling out. When the need arises, with the whip on the outside, the horse is encouraged to step over more, or the whip is placed on the inside to improve the forward drive.

With a young horse it is better to carry out the half pass starting from a turn and adding the half pass onto it. The horse's body must stay parallel to the wall of the arena with a good contact and definite bend in the direction of the movement, and a distinct elevation of the forehand. As soon as the horse and rider have been able to reduce the size of the turning circle with the half pass, the lesson is extended and ridden from the midline into a half pass. Once the horse is skilled enough to perform a flowing half pass on short sections of the arena, the exercise can be developed from one side of the arena to the other. An exercise I can recommend is: volte-half pass-volte, and always only a few steps.

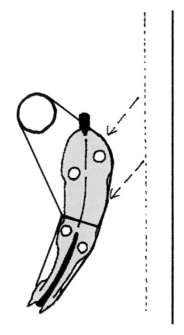

Half pass on long reins.

This exercise can be executed on long reins in all the basic gaits and can also be ridden. There are a few points that have to be observed: at the walk it must be remembered that this is the gait with the least impulsion and that the half pass can be easier performed in gaits with more impulsion. The most uncomplicated gait for all the lateral work is the trot. The canter may have a bigger capacity for impulsion, but it is often more difficult to achieve collection in canter than in the trot. Many horses will simply run off the first time the half pass is requested at the canter, in such situations the trainer must concentrate more on the collection of the canter first.

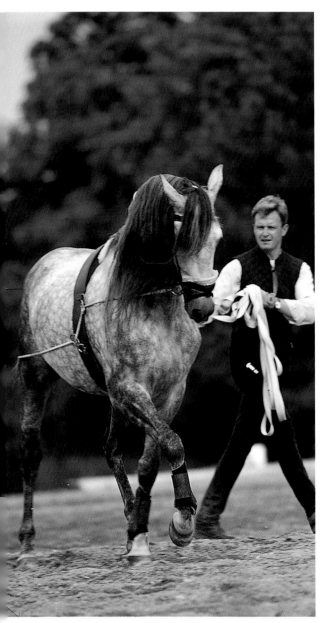

Trot half pass on long reins

Exercises such as trot or walk transitions as well as halts and then canter directly from the standstill are amongst those that will help this situation. When working with long reins, it is generally better to wait until the horse has mastered collection in the canter before attempting it. A further variation to the trot half pass is to interrupt the half pass by moving on a straight line for a few strides and then resume the half pass once more. The exercise can be further enhanced when a few strides on the straight line are lengthened, perhaps to medium trot. Another excellent exercise is to interrupt the half pass with walk or halt transitions, these additions have a similar gymnastic value to the shoulder in for they enhance the stepping under of the legs and carrying more weight on the hindlegs. The trot after the halt should start off with a few straight steps and afterwards continue in the half pass to avoid the possible loss of impulsion and rhythm. When performing these exercises, an important detail to keep an eye on is the outside rein.

An additional exercise to improve the half pass is as follows: you start a volte on the second corner of the short side of the arena. From the corner on the long side of the arena, begin a half pass that travels to approximately 8 metres before the opposite wall of the arena, where a volte will produce the half pass going in the other direction. This exercise can be continued until the trainer is completely satisfied.

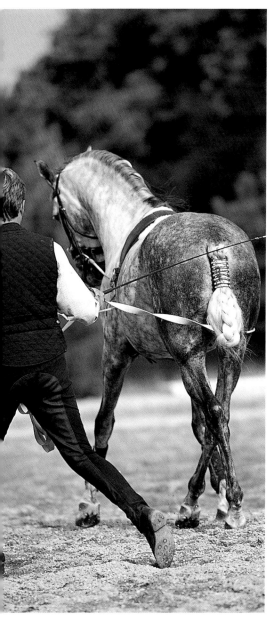

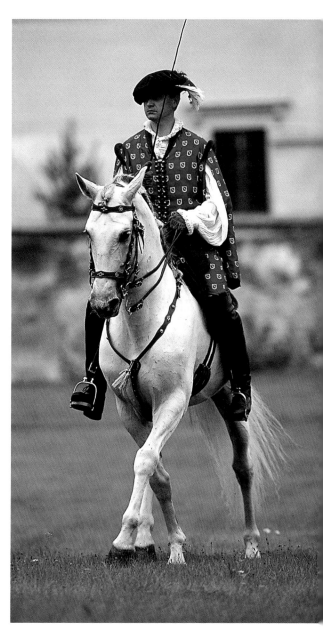

Half pass left: good contact and bend of the horse

Half pass right. Please note: good seat and gaze direction from the rider, contact, bend and cross-over from the attentive horse

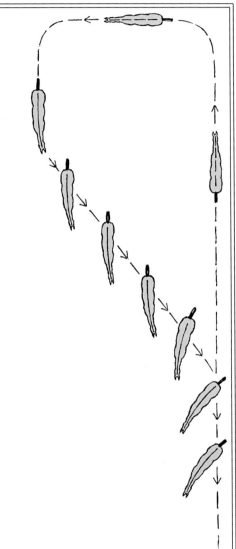

Transition from half pass to renvers

The trainer can work both on the inside as well as on the outside of the horse, although he must stay closer to the horse on the outside but will then be more exposed to the danger of the horse's hindlegs.

For the most part it is more desirable for the trainer to move on the horse's inside with a little distance between him and the horse, especially as this is also the more straightforward way to guide the horse in travers. The trainer will definitely need the assistance of a driving whip in order to reach the side of the horse that is turned away from him. This obviously demands some skill and practice from the trainer on long reins.

THE FULL PASS

The full pass is all about moving sideways with no forward movement involved. This is only performed under the rider and is only mentioned here to complete the picture. This lateral movement comes from the military school and functions as an aid to rectify the position the rider has relative to other riders in a formation. In the Vaquero training this is a technique that is still used, it is even expected in their assessment. The Vaqueros make use of the full pass when they have to open and close gates on the pastures without having to get off their horses. The full pass can only be executed in the correct way when it is performed from a halt. The horse is asked to take a step. As soon as the foot of the horse leaves the ground, the inside rein leads the forehand to the side where the pass is to be directed, while the outside rein disallows any forward movement. The rider's inside leg prevents any step backwards and requires the corresponding bend.

The rider's outside leg lies behind the girth and drives the horse to the side. The full pass is terminated again in a halt.

FAULTS IN TRAVERS AND HALF PASS, AND THE CORRECTION

Hindquarters leading:

This is the fault that appears when the comprehension of the sideways movement is incorrect. This fault is for the most part accompanied by an obvious loss of impulsion. A short break in the half pass by moving on a straight line and a noticeable forward push of the horse's shoulder with the outside rein will normally help to rectify this situation. This fault chiefly comes about under the rider and seldom occurs on long reins.

Insufficient cross-over of the legs:

There are two sources of this fault, and one of them should not be considered a fault. Young horses will seldom achieve significant cross-over of their legs, this is mainly due to the level of education and they can, with the correct training, attain a more superior cross-over in time. The second source of this fault is, as so often, the loss of impulsion. A distinct driving inside aid and light hand will resolve this matter.

Too much sideways movement:

This happens when the horse has too much movement to the side as opposed to for-

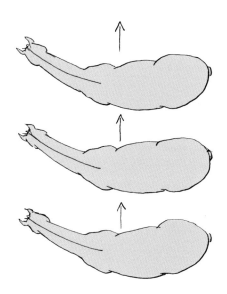

Full pass

ward movement; in other words the horse withdraws from the movement by means of too much sideways movement and too little forward movement. A definite help from the whip, together with the rider's leg, can remedy this by triggering more forward movement. Unfortunately, it is often not enough as a remedy. When this is the case, the trainer can interrupt the half pass with a few straight steps, as described above and then continue with the half pass in the same direction or change the direction of the half pass back in the direction of the wall. The horse will pay more attention to the rider's leg with this last exercise, as it will not be able to anticipate the direction of the half pass.

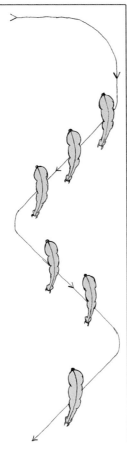

A further exercise to develop suppleness to combat problems with bend and contact: half pass-leg yield-half pass

Faults and obstructions caused by the seat of the rider:

· The rider sits with his weight in the opposite direction to the movement.
· The rider does not look into the direction of the movement.
· The rider's inside hip falls in or the outside hip falls out.

· The inside hand crosses over the withers of the horse.
· The rider's shoulder is not parallel to the shoulder of the horse; the hips are not parallel to the horse's.

All the above faults of the seat of the rider have a direct and evident influence over the movement of the horse.

There is considerably more I could say about lateral work – it could fill another book of its own – with the whip on the outside but I think I have pointed out the most important fundamental features in the foregoing pages.

THE HORSE READY FOR THE DOUBLE BRIDLE

At this stage of its training the horse becomes accustomed to the double bridle as well. The double bridle is the term for the bridle that has two bits, namely a curb bit with a bridoon. At this stage the horse must be capable of a medium degree of collection. This way of going will ensure that there is no unfavourable result for the horse to be ridden in a double bridle. The horse must be familiarised with the effect of the curb bit. However, it should not constantly be ridden on the curb but mainly on the bridoon, which acts like a snaffle bit.

As a rule, the horse should be worked in the double bridle two or three times a week. The horse must never be ridden on the curb bit simply for the reason that the rider cannot create the desired frame of the horse without it.

Every curb bit, be it as mild or soft as possible, nonetheless has a lever action that depends on the proportion between the lengths of the upper and lower parts of the cheeks of the curb and the effect it has on the bars of the mouth. The curb chain will add extra pressure to the chin of the horse as well. The narrower the curb chain and the fewer links it has, the more severe the action. The application of the curb chain can be regulated and leather and rubber covers can be employed to lessen the severity of the action.

The horse is now ridden in a working tempo in all the basic gaits on long curved and straight lines in order to get it accustomed to the double bridle. The horse is requested to bend and stretch and all the while the curb bit is not touched, while the horse is ridden only with the use of the bridoon. In the interest of safety, the curb chain is left out completely or attached only loosely. The curb chain is only linked into the correct tightness after many free and easy sessions of riding with the rider's hands soft and almost passive and the horse stepping under his body weight with satisfactory impulsion. The cheeks of the curb should create an angle of 40 to 34 degrees with the mouth when the rein is taken up. Only after the horse accepts the effect of the double bridle through further free and

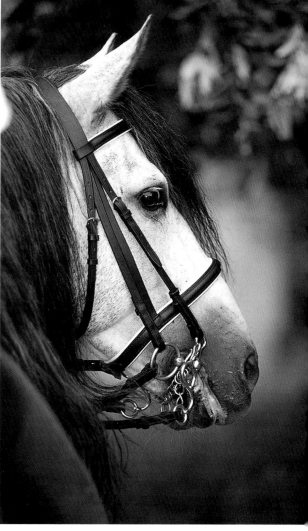

Double bridle with a Portuguese S-curb

easy sessions can the rider request the first lesson of contact with the relevant amount of collection that accompanies it.

There are very many severe bits that have been invented since the horse started to serve man. This undeniably points to the fact that man is a "worker with the hand", and that, per se, has nothing to do with

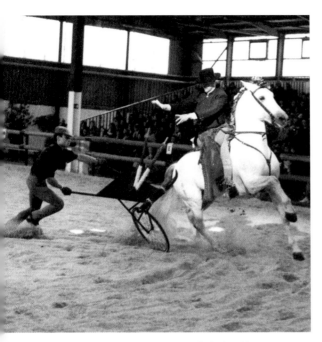

With the refinement of the aids the hand becomes superfluous: Cartucho under the author in a simulated bull fight.

the classical art of riding. In this day and age there are still instruments of torture being invented, which include bicycle chains in the mouths of horses.

Man has always tried to retaliate with technique, to even the score, for his inadequate riding capability and lack of understanding for the nature of the art of riding. This does not mean, however, that the rider must take revenge with the curb and become a persecutor. Riding on the curb only is best left to the masters who truly have independent and balanced seats. Riding on the curb only with both reins in one hand and the whip held pointing skywards in the other hand is the ultimate perfection

of subtle aids. The hand is held completely quiet over the mane and produces only the smallest of impulses that are invisible to the onlooker. The horse is ridden with only the seat of the rider and the slightest aids from the legs. The maximum expression of this refinement is visible in the bullfight on horseback, where the reins are tied to the rider's belt and the horse reacts merely to the weight aids from the rider.

It is extremely important not to ride the horse on the double bridle too soon, for this will reinforce all the faults in the training immediately. There are frequently faults in the gaits or rein contact in horses that were put in double bridles too soon, before they have achieved the necessary maturity.

There are three basic methods to control the reins of the double bridle:

· Two on each side: curb rein under the ring finger, bridoon rein under the little finger – the most conventional technique.
· Three to one: the bridoon rein of the right side is held under the left ring finger, the left hand holds also holds the left bridoon rein under the little finger, the left curb rein under the ring finger and under the middle finger the right curb rein. This manner of control dates back to the time when people fought on horseback, for it is easier to have the reins in one hand and thus leave the other free to brandish a weapon. In the Spanish Riding School tradition still allows

the riders to ride in this way.

· The Fillis way: this instructor rode with the reins of the curb under the little finger and the reins of the bridoon over the index finger.

The method of controlling the reins of the double bridle is partly one of personal preference and partly one of specific objectives. The 2:2 method is the most straightforward, 3:1 is used when the curb must be particularly quiet and equal on both reins and no one-sided influence of the curb is desired on the mouth of the horse. The Fillis method has the advantage that the influence of the curb and the bridoon can be administered separately in the exact amounts required.

The use of the double bridle is almost exclusively kept for riding. On the long reins the double bridle is sporadically used by selected trainers on the Iberian peninsula and they will then employ the different methods of controlling the reins described in the paragraphs above.

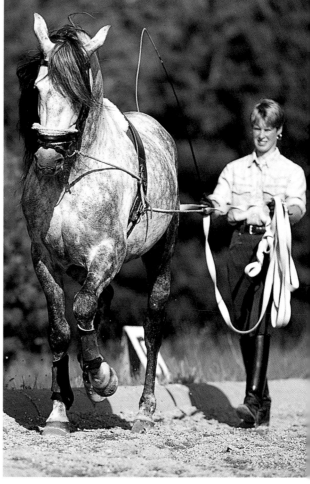

The request for the piaffe on the long rein

PIAFFE

As soon as the lateral work is so far advanced that the horse can execute the movements without difficulties, the training can be increased in intensity and can build up to the gaits of the high school movements. These consist of the collected trot, collected canter, piaffe and passage. The piaffe, the trot in one place, is distin-guished through further flexion of the hocks and elevation of the forehand that is the result of pure collection. The rhythm of the piaffe is somewhat slower than the rhythm of the natural trot of the horse. The horse moves with powerful springy steps in diagonal pairs and carries his body weight more on the hindquarters. The

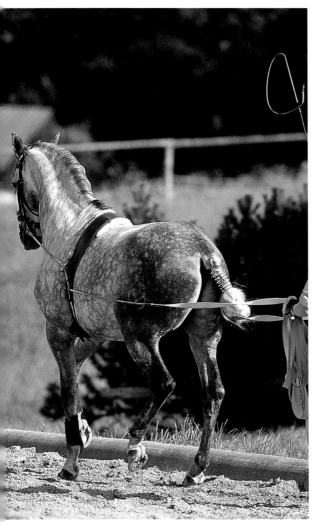

Julepe in the transition to the piaffe

steps under his body weight, and is not artificially produced.

This lesson has enormous gymnastic value through the request for additional weight bearing on the hindquarters. There are two basic possibilities from which to develop the piaffe, namely from the walk and the trot. When do you use which option? The piaffe is requested from the walk if the horse has a more explosive or nervous personality, but it is asked from the trot when the horse is a more lethargic type. In support of the piaffe on the long rein, a driving whip is used at first and with it the dock of the tail is tapped, as much as is necessary and as little as possible! The first exercise is to walk behind the horse on the track of the arena and repeat the transition of the halt from the trot. During the exercise the distances between the transitions must be shortened (three or four steps) until the horse shows some definite attempts towards the piaffe as is often the case in talented horses. When the horse accepts this exercise without anxiety, the next introductory exercise can be attempted. In the trot-halt transitions, a rein-back is incorporated (three to four steps) and the trot is demanded from the rein-back without a halt. Both these preliminary exercises must be commenced on the track of the arena but should sooner rather than later be undertaken away from the track as well. Attempts to do the piaffe should already be quite obvious in these lessons. Now the time is ripe to shorten the steps even fur-

horse in piaffe must always place the feet one hoof print in front of the other, in other words there must be a predisposition for slight forward movement. The exception is of course the horse between the pillars. The high school jumps such as the levade and capriole arise from the piaffe at a later stage. The elevation of the forehand arises from the enhanced way the horse ther. Doing these exercises on both reins should be a matter of course, although exercises should be carried out slightly more on the better rein while the exercise on the more difficult rein must every so often be executed in such a kind way that the horse does not realise it soon enough to be able to resist the trainer!

Do not expect too much of the horse at the first attempt: 1 centimetre per day adds up to 3 metres at the end of the year!

When the horse is overtaxed in the beginning, the setbacks are harsh at a later stage. The actual piaffe exercise should not be more than ten minutes, for it is extremely tiring for the horse, especially in the beginning. If the horse is additionally schooled on free lines in the introductory exercises, the piaffe will soon be successful and contribute to more expression and freedom of the steps. The attempt at piaffe on the free line should in the beginning definitely consist of only a few steps and increase the quantity of steps gradually. The piaffe on free lines should, however, be started in close approximation to the track and the distance extended little by little, so that the horse can grow accustomed to it at a slow pace.

It is recommended to commence the piaffe from a shoulder in or travers if the horse is exceedingly responsive or nervous. This approach requires a great deal of sensitivity from the trainer for the horse's rhythm. The following assignment can be quite helpful in this scenario: start the

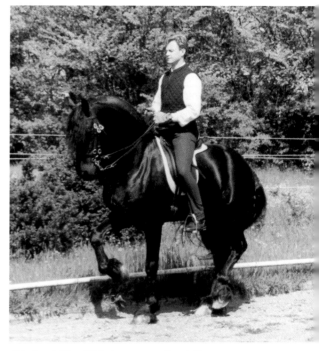

Friesian stallion Wiebe in an expressive piaffe

shoulder in from a volte on the long side of the arena and slowly shorten the steps of the shoulder in with the use of half-halts on the outside rein. The preliminary exercise of trot-walk transitions done earlier in the shoulder in will be extremely useful and make the exercise straightforward. It is of paramount significance that the impulsion does not get lost in the exercises for piaffe and that the horse does not lose the forward movement in the process. The forward motion of the horse can not only be stimulated, but also tested in transitions from the piaffe into trot. If the horse does not stride out of the piaffe with enthusiasm, the problem is an obvious loss of impulsion and forward movement. On the basis of all the different examples of how to develop the piaffe, it is evident that the one exercise will gain something from the others as well. This is the only way forward to gymnastic training, not via artificial routes.

At the same time as the horse starts to shorten his strides, the trainer can in addition begin to tap the hindleg of the horse with a whip, namely every time a leg touches the ground, it is tapped with the whip. The different positions the horse can be touched with the whipare explainded in the chapter "Training in hand according to the Viennese school".

A further way of working out the piaffe is to shorten the strides in the half pass: collected trot coming out of the corner – change the rein – half pass to the track and in the process shortening the stride – at the wall, trot to keep the impulsion and in the next corner repeat the whole exercise. As soon as possible the piaffe must be demanded on free lines and without the preceding lateral gaits. It can take up to a year, in some cases even longer, before the piaffe is matured enough and the horse can actually perform the piaffe under the weight of the rider. If the trainer makes as little use of the whip as possible, the ridden piaffe will require considerably less effort to perform. When the horse is adept enough to execute some piaffe steps under the weight of a passive rider, the time has finally come to encourage the completion of the piaffe under the rider. A number of

horses can perform the piaffe under the rider parallel to the work on the long rein, but others are completely traumatised by the simultaneous demand. Observe the horse in detail and it is better to start the piaffe under saddle at a later stage rather than too early, for once the horse has acquired faults such as losing rhythm or hurried steps, they are seldom, if ever, properly corrected. As is the case in most situations, it is better to avoid faults through thorough compassionate action than to rectify them later at a cost.

More detail on the work on piaffe under the rider will be available in the chapter "Training in hand according to the Viennese school". From the moment the horse can perform the piaffe in a skilful and correct manner, the trainer can refine the piaffe with the lessons used in the Iberian and Viennese techniques, more of which in the appropriate chapters.

FAULTS IN THE PIAFFE, AND THEIR CORRECTION

All the faults in the piaffe are easier to correct in hand than under the rider.

Rocking from side to side:

The impulsion of the horse must be improved. Transitions from trot to piaffe and from piaffe into trot the moment the horse commences with this, is useful to combat the fault. Having said that, there are still horses that never completely let go of this imperfection. The correction of this fault must be without a rider in the begin-

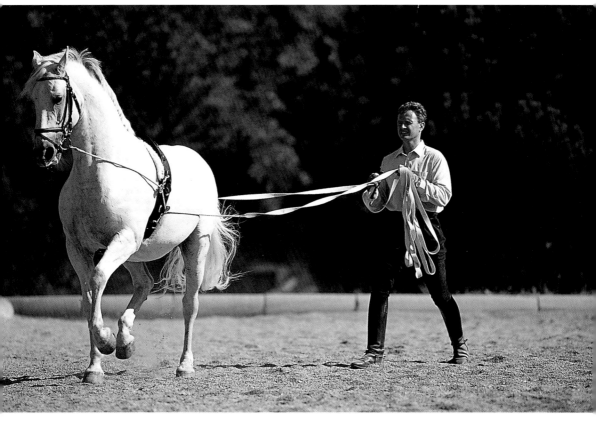

Maestoso Ancona in piaffe on a free line.

ning. Only once there is a distinct improvement, can this be practised under the rider. To summarise, it can be said: if the piaffe is properly performed from the start and the impulsion not lost for a moment, this fault will not come about.

Faulty rhythm in the piaffe:

This fault can also be rectified with definite forward driving of the horse. Every occasion the horse falls into this trap, the trot must be employed to drive it on, only

to change into the piaffe again. The rhythmical tapping of the horse's legs is mostly not enough to correct this fault; on occasion it even worsens it!

Hindquarters trailing:

This fault almost always comes to pass when the horse first learned the passage and then had to develop the piaffe from it.

The piaffe is then nothing more than rhythmical steps in one spot without flexion of the hocks. These horses will mostly be artificially elevated which means they will hollow their backs as well. This makes the piaffe not only incorrect, but damaging, and the correction of it almost impossible. In this set of circumstances I would start the piaffe from the beginning, as if the horse had never performed it before. Occasionally in this way the piaffe can be improved upon. The accomplishment of the correction depends greatly on the length of time the fault has existed.

Forming a V:

The horse's hindquarters and the forehand draw closer to each other and superficially this gives the impression of collection. With closer inspection it will be detected that the poll is not the highest point any more, but the horse has lightened the load on the hindquarters and is therefore on the forehand.

The forehand is moving closer to the hindquarters and not the other way round as should be the case. This mistake is seen often but it is relatively straightforward to rectify. A distinct transition into working or even medium trot and then again the transition back to piaffe will lift the horse and the impulsion and elevation created should be kept in the piaffe. When this fault occurs, it is suggested that, at least for a while, the piaffe should not be performed from the walk, but only from the trot. As soon as the error slips in, the horse must immediately be requested to trot, even better if it can be done before the fault even arises.

Accelerated piaffe:

This error is mostly seen in extremely sensitive and nervous horses. There are two possible techniques to correct this, but both demand a great deal of compassion from the trainer. The first technique, on the long rein, is slowly and carefully to request the piaffe from the halt or the walk without touching the horse too much with the whip, and as soon as the horse descends into the fault again to return to the walk or halt again. The horse must then be calmed down if necessary and the whole process started from the halt or walk yet again: an arduous and patience-demanding task! The second, even more difficult adjustment is accomplished between the pillars and will be discussed in some detail in the corresponding chapter.

PASSAGE

The passage can now be developed out of the correct piaffe. The passage should never be requested before the piaffe, for the result is almost always an appalling piaffe and repeated passage-like steps that the horse will use to resist in other lessons. It is equally important to engender a feeling of certainty that the horse is confident in the lateral work before even attempting to teach it the passage.

The passage is another a movement that was taken from the horse's natural flamboyance. It is the stallion's way of impress-

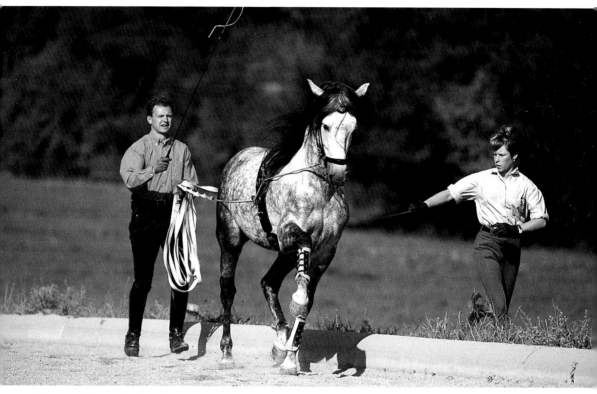

Julepe on the long rein: lesson in passage

ing the mares in the wild and makes it seem larger than life to any possible rival in order to avoid a fight for the position of leader in the pecking order. This should not be confused with the high stepping trot that horses perform when they are excited. From the point of the horse's psychology the passage cannot be demanded through brute force, for the expression of the passage will certainly be lost. The passage must have the sensation of lightness, yes, of flying, as if the horse is not touching the ground. The horse must not look as if it was forced and threatened into doing it. Once the piaffe is perfected, the

passage is not a problem, for most of the time the horse will offer the movement spontaneously. If the piaffe was achieved with the use of the Iberian and Viennese techniques, the passage will, if truth be told, happen particularly free from stress. The trainer should then return to the work on long reins, for it will be easier to keep the impulsion going in this manner.

The horse is requested to perform the piaffe on the long side of the arena and is offered more freedom without changing the rhythm, collection or elevation. The trainer expects only one, two or even three steps in the beginning and extensively praises the understood it and can at any time perform the lesson when requested. Horses that have a natural talent for passage will easily enough learn the passage in this way.

If the horse does not have such a natural ability, another means of encouragement must be called upon: the front legs must be tapped with the whip. The exact points of reference are available in the chapter "Training in hand according to the Viennese school". A normal whip can be utilised or even a bamboo reed that, when correctly employed, does not injure the horse, but the amount of noise it produces when the trainer taps the legs of the horse should be adequate encouragement.

If the horse is not showing any reaction to the tapping on the legs even when it is accompanied with the desired amount of impulsion, it might be that the passage is requested too early or that the horse is not ready for the passage yet, or even that the horse does not have the ability to do passage at all, which can also be possible. When the horse demonstrates no sign of cadenced steps or his movement even becomes frantic, it might well be an indication of asking too much too soon. In order to develop the passage through the tapping of the front legs, it is necessary to have a helper who is capable either of using the whip or managing the long reins. When using the whip, it is extremely important to find the right moment: the moment is as soon as the horse lifts the front leg off the ground and while this leg is still on its way

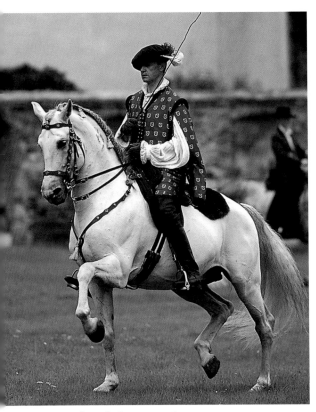

Cartucho in an expressive passage.

horse when it is successful. Of the utmost important and probably the decisive factor is the interaction between driving aids (voice, whip) and the restraining aids (hand).

The passage is, as discussed in the previous chapter, the gait with the most cadence that the horse can be taught. An enormous quantity of balance and weight-carrying ability of the hindquarters, with elevation, is required to develop the passage in the correct manner into an impressive way of going. The lesson previously described must be repeated until the horse has up. As a rule it is a great deal more difficult to manage the long reins for this is where the impulsion and collection of the horse must be maintained! The more accomplished the horse is, the more steps are likely.

Parallel to the work in hand, the passage must be promoted under the rider as well until the horse can maintain the passage through turns, circles and even voltes. The most talented horses can even achieve a half pass passage in a zigzag pattern. The passage is naturally a great deal more difficult and the trainer must expect only a few steps in the beginning. Once the horse is ready to commence the passage under the rider, the horse should be allowed additional freedom as was done on the long reins, while the helper aids with the tapping of the whip on the front legs of the horse. The hand of the rider stays firm and develops some tension. If the tension in the hand becomes too much and the rider puts too much weight in the horse's mouth, the horse will consider it a half-halt and change to a halt or relocate to the piaffe once more.

Both the legs of the rider must enclose the horse; the rider must obtain the impression that he can physically lift the horse from the ground with his legs. If the horse grows to be restless, it is usually a good idea to halt, if the horse pulls, halt in any case, ask the horse to rein back without engaging in battle and repeat the passage all over again. If the horse loses tension and collection it is generally better to

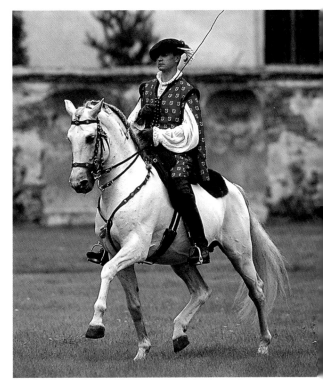

Transition passage-lengthened trot.

return to the piaffe yet again. There are of course exceptions to every rule, but as we all know, the exceptions make the rule. The work in the passage must by and large be composed and may under no circumstances agitate or excite the horse.

FAULTS IN THE PASSAGE, AND THE CORRECTION

As is the case with the piaffe, the faults in the passage can develop from incorrect training or conformation, and these faults can be difficult to rectify and in severe cases even impossible to correct. The accomplishment of the correction will depend on the length of time the fault existed.

Swaying passage:

This fault has already been mentioned in the piaffe. Most of the time this error comes about through the seat of the rider. The rider frequently thinks that he should travel to extremes with the movement and in doing this will cause the swaying motion in the horse. In this instance the cause, namely the seat of the rider, must firstly be corrected. The second cause of the problem is that the hindquarters were not quite strong enough at the commencement of the lessons in passage. Improvement of this problem is never easy and can be exceedingly lengthy. As with many things in the art of riding it must be rectified with the increase of impulsion. The passage is asked with a reduced amount of collection but more forward movement. Transitions from passage into lengthened trot and back into the passage can be of enormous help in this case. An additional correction that can be employed is the shoulder in in the passage.

These lessons require a particularly sensitive rider for the lateral aids must be given only delicately in order to prevent the horse from falling back into trot. The rider should pay special attention to his seat, whether he is straight and in balance, neither in front of nor behind the movement and without clutching onto the reins. All of these features can instigate the swaying of the horse and the passage will unquestionably lose its grandeur and expression.

Loss of rhythm:

This is in principle the same fault as already described in the piaffe and therefore the same corrections will apply. The trainer will rectify the error here through driving the horse forward and through transitions into the trot. This fault will mainly be noticed if the horse feels overtaxed, for that reason the trainer must ask for only a few strides in the correction and increase the demand little by little every time.

Stiff back and trailing hindquarters:

This will almost certainly be the fault if the horse runs away from the movement. The cause is often, but not always, a matter of overtaxing the horse. It can quite often also be a strong hand from the rider that causes it. The response should be: recognise the cause, remove the cause and correct the effect. The correction follows from many halts and then requesting the passage again, both on the long reins and under the rider. If the horse shows extreme trailing of the hindquarters when it halts, the rectification might be to perform a rein back from the halt and then to request the passage directly from the rein back. A light and sensitive hand from the rider is especially essential in the correction of this fault. Remember that!

Letting the forelegs hang:

Some horses, very often the sport horses, leave the forelegs dangling without any expression. This fault is the result of too little collection. It can either be that the horse is not capable of higher collection due to the build of his body, or the horse never learnt

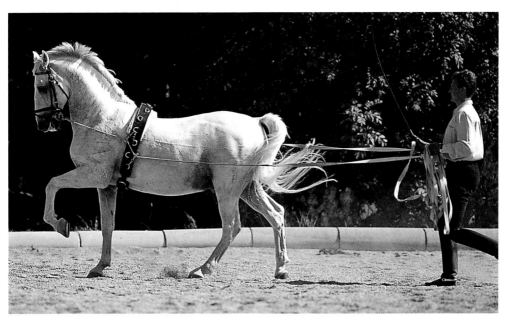

Maestoso Ancona in a straight canter on the long reins

the amount of collection required for the passage. The answer to this problem is to return to the piaffe once more and to go to work yet again on the collection of the horse. After that we return to the passage where the horse's front legs as well as the back legs should be tapped. A higher and more rounded action of the legs is achieved when the coronet band of the foot is tapped with the bamboo reed.

CANTER AND COUNTER CANTER

CANTER

The canter demands a lot of fitness on the part of the trainer and a horse that is capable of doing an extremely short canter,

which, after the learning of the piaffe, should be no problem. An excellent way to achieve canter on the long reins, is to request a shoulder in right before the corner of the school.

With the help of the trainer's voice, a half-halt on the outside rein and a tap with the whip just behind the girth on the inside, the horse then canters on. After some trot-canter-trot transitions on the circle, the same exercise is demanded on straight lines, and also in the volte and then incorporates the transitions into walk and the halt. The transitions to walk and halt are prepared with half-halts on the outside rein, performed in the rhythm of the canter at exactly the moment the outside hindfoot leaves the ground. The half-halts are performed two or three canter strides before the downward transition is required to allow the horse to shorten the canter strides and to take more weight on the hindquarters. Then it is straightforward to carry out the transition. The next step is lateral work in the canter.

The first of these is the plié-canter, or the canter shoulder in. The collection of the canter can also additionally be improved with this lesson. In principle the aids for the canter shoulder in on the long reins and under the rider are the same as for the shoulder in at the trot. The horse is also driven sideways and forward with the rhythm of the movement. The outside rein is of more significance due to the increase in impulsion. If the outside rein is absent the horse will only run away with his head turned sideways. It is therefore of immense importance to pay attention to the outside aids.

COUNTER CANTER

In the counter canter the aids are simply the exact opposite to those for the normal canter. While the rider's inside leg, slightly behind the girth, confirms the aid for the counter canter, the outside leg will promote the lively jump of every stride. The horse is bent to the outside and has the contact in that way as well, the outside rein leads the horse along the wall, the inside rein restricts the amount of bend to the outside and supports the outside rein. The counter canter on the long rein is required only once the horse has under-

stood the counter canter under the rider. The aids for the counter canter on the long reins are the same as for the normal canter, only the other way round.

There is a practical way to teach the horse the counter canter. By far the easiest way is to ride a simple serpentine and ask for an outside (counter) canter when the horse is at its furthest away from the track. Now the horse is taken back to the track and must canter around the first corner. If this is successful, the rider gives the horse a half halt into the trot before the next corner and praises the horse. This is repeated once more and then attempted on the other rein. Once the horse is secure in this exercise, the rider can ask the horse to counter canter around both corners. If there are any problems in retaining the counter canter through the corner, the first point to pay attention to is to ensure that the corners are not ridden too deep and also to start the canter just before the corner, for as a rule, the quality of the collection is best at the beginning of the canter. In a large arena, for example a jumping arena, there is another way to work at the counter canter. The rider rides the horse on a very big circle (about 30 metres in diameter), leads the horse into a volte to the outside and asks for the canter, only to return to the circle in a counter canter. Whenever the horse shows signs that it has difficulty in persisting with the counter canter, the rider takes the horse back into a volte to the outside and then returns to the circle once more in a counter canter.

FAULTS IN THE COUNTER CANTER, AND THEIR CORRECTION

Cantering on two tracks is a severe mistake and must immediately receive the attention it deserves by straightening the horse with the help of both hands.

This mistake often occurs because the rider demanded too much collection at the beginning. More impulsion, sometimes even a few lengthened canter strides, will often resolve this matter.

A further fault is, of course, the horse changing the canter lead without the aid of the rider. On the whole this happens owing to the fact that the rider expected too much from the beginning. The rider should reduce the demand on the horse!

SIMPLE CHANGE

As soon as the horse has mastered the lesson of counter canter without any problems, the next exercise it has to learn is the simple change. The definition of the simple change is the half-halt of the horse from the canter into the walk and, depending on the skill of the horse, after a few steps in the walk, recommencing the canter on the other rein. This transition, whose fluid and smooth implementation is the prerequisite for the flying change that will come later on, should present the horse with no difficulties at this level of training. The first step is to teach the horse to canter from the walk. In order for this to

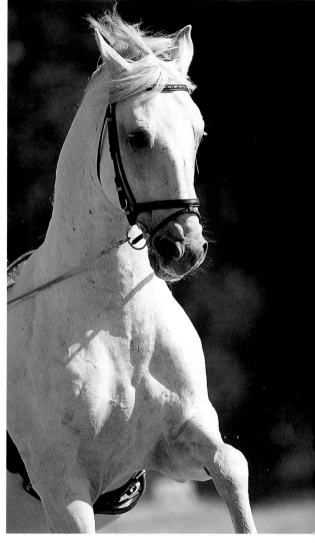

Elevated, dynamic canter on the long rein

come about, the walk must be more collected, elevated and hold more cadence. The steps become shorter, the print of the hindfoot does not reach that of the forefoot. At this stage it is important to pay attention to the purity of the walk, and the purity of the gaits in general at this high attempted from the canter.

In order to achieve this, the horse must be further shortened and collected for one or two canter strides. In the beginning this will be more comfortable when the horse is ridden in a decreasing circle. The horse is shortened for a few strides, on the long reins this should cause no problems on a decreasing circle, and the horse is then allowed to canter on with greater strides without the half-halt into the walk. This is repeated on both reins until the horse shortens and collects itself without any trouble. Naturally this exercise is repeated under the rider as well. The significant aid, both on the long rein and under saddle is the forward driving aid and this must always be predominant. Under the rider this is the inside leg and on the long rein this is the whip carried slightly higher behind the horse. The outside rein of the rider as well as the long rein controls the tempo without tightening. At this point the trainer must attempt to half-halt the horse once or twice, from two shortened canter strides, into the walk transition. Under the rider this half-halt is influenced by breathing out deeply, which will have a positive effect on the seat of the rider.

If the transition is successful, a medium walk of at least six steps is performed. Once again the walk must be carefully examined for purity and appropriately sized steps. As soon as the transition from the canter to the walk is successful on both reins, the trainer can request the horse to canter again after a

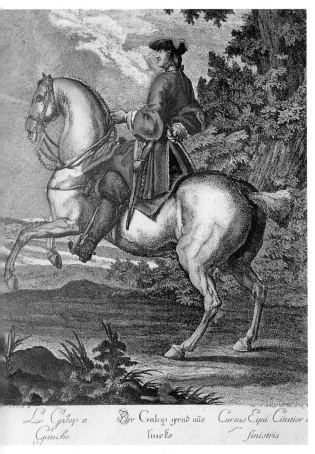

Baroque portrayal of the canter, an engraving by Ridinger

level of training! The walk is collected for a few paces only; as soon as the steps of the walk become spoiled, the rider must immediately move on to medium walk.

To keep the walk pure and nevertheless prepare the horse for a canter, it is recommended to perform the shoulder in at the walk and to present the initiating canter aids from the shoulder in at the walk. Once the horse has learnt to canter correctly from the walk without delay on the canter aids, the half-halt to the walk can be few metres of walk. Once this is satisfactorily achieved, the trainer can then request a simple change of the canter.

This change should nonetheless have an interval of at least seven walk strides, showing the purity of the walk. The walk between the two canters must always have an uneven number of strides; this will instigate the correct lead on the new rein without the horse having to attempt an extra short stride before the strike-off, so do count with your horse! The simple change is still performed from the decreasing circle while the horse only rehearses the half-halt into the walk from the canter on the long reins.

An excellent technique to half-halt the horse into the walk is to request the walk two or three canter strides from the commencement of the canter. The horse will pass on the collection from the canter that is ultimately required for the walk. Numerous repetitions of this exercise will strengthen the objective of the half-halt to walk in the horse's mind. Later on the exercise of the simple change is requested on a straight line, which is substantially more difficult for the horse.

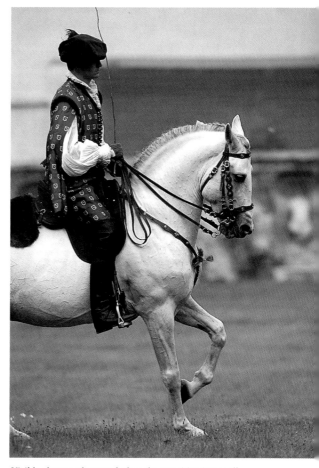

Visibly shortened canter before the transition into walk

FAULTS IN THE SIMPLE CANTER CHANGE, AND THEIR CORRECTION
Falling on the forehand in the walk:
The horse is not sufficiently prepared for the lesson. The horse must be noticeably more collected before the transition, meaning at least one or two canter strides must be shortened beforehand. As correction, the phase of shortening must be more pronounced and an extra canter stride can be added. If needs be, the trainer must return to the exercise already described where the circle is reduced. On the long reins the transition is demanded at a higher tempo, the horse perceptibly shortened and the trainer attempts to carry the impulsion from the canter into the walk.

The walk is not pure or is too fast:

This fault is seen predominantly in temperamental horses, but its cause frequently is due to a strong hand from the rider or trainer on the lunge. There are two possible techniques to rectify a walk with steps that are too quick:

· The trainer can request many more steps in the walk, until the horse is calmer, before attempting the canter on the other rein.

· The trainer asks for a halt after the transition into walk, lets the horse do a few strides of rein back and then continues forward in the walk. This is repeated until the horse calms down sufficiently.

An impure footfall or even a pace is always caused by the shortcomings of the rider's hand. There are, of course, horses that are inclined naturally to pace. If the trainer stays attentive in the schooling of the horse, the incorrect gait of the pace can be avoided altogether. As soon as the horse falls into the pace after the walk transition, the trainer must give with the hand and allow the horse to stretch into a ground-covering walk. Under no circumstances may the horse be allowed to canter before the walk is not pure. If this fault cannot be corrected with the give of the hand, the shortcoming must be sought in the schooling that preceded this. The correction to this fault can be lengthy and will mostly revert to the foundation of schooling. One technique to attempt the correction of this fault is to move into a shoulder in straight after the

transition into walk. The trainer must work on the basics, the horse should stay supple, relaxed and composed. No collected walk must be required in the basic training! A phase of tautness must be followed by a phase of relaxation,

The walk transition is stretched out:

When there is an interruption to the flow of the movement it is mostly due to the hard hand of the rider or the fact that the upper body of the rider has fallen forward or the driving aids are not dedicated enough. The hand of the rider should stay relaxed, without becoming rigid and give in the transition to the walk, the leg must stay on the horse to administer the driving aids should the need arise and the upper body must stay upright. The hand must be equally kind and giving on the long reins while the driving aids should be the prevailing ones. This fault will often be accompanied by the horse becoming heavy on the forehand.

The walk transition is stretched out:

When we speak of a walk transition as stretched out, it means the horse was not collected enough and did not sit on his haunches to move into the walk from the canter and the whole incident has the look of being blurred and not clear cut. The correction for this fault is the same as with the horse on the forehand. The horse must be better prepared to perform this transition, the trainer requests another shorter canter stride before the transition into walk or failing that, must return to the exercise where the circle is reduced.

No canter on the aids or delayed reaction to the aids:

The most important factor in such a situation is that the horse must be better prepared for the canter. The horse's attention is drawn to the aids for the canter. This is the case under the rider as well as on the long reins.

If this does not improve the jump into canter or make it easier, the trainer can demand a few steps in rein back and from there give the canter aids once more.

CANTER PIROUETTE

The canter pirouette is the smallest turn the horse can make in a canter. The correct implementation of the canter pirouette depends to a great degree on a canter with a

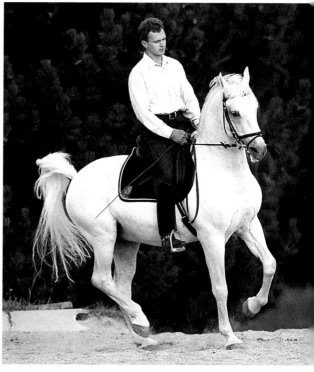

Maestoso Ancona in the right canter pirouette

copious amount of impulsion. There are half (180 degrees), three-quarters (270 degrees) and full (360 degrees) pirouettes. Horses that have immense athletic abilities can even perform double pirouettes. The half pirouette consists of three to four canter jumps, the three-quarter pirouette consists of four to six canter jumps and the full pirouette consists of six to eight canter jumps. Besides the classical pirouette just described, there is also the faster pirouette of the Iberian cowboys, the so-called Vaquero-pirouette, where the number of canter jumps is halved.

The pirouette comprises uniform, rhythmical canter jumps around the hindquarters where the inside leg creates the midpoint. The pirouette can be ridden from the renvers, half pass and the track. The goal should always be to ride the pirouette from the simple track, for this is the correct way according to the old classical technique. Developing the pirouette from the renvers is the best way to teach the horse, the pirouette from the half pass promotes the horse's attentiveness to the aids. No matter how the pirouette is started, according to the classical way it must end in the same manner: when commenced from the half pass it must end in the half pass, from the renvers back into the renvers, from the simple track to the simple track!

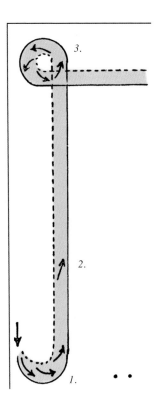

1. Passade 2. Renvers 3. Pirouette in the corner

The aids for the pirouette under the rider:

the inside rein will lead the horse into the turn while the inside leg on the girth drives increasingly in order to maintain the impulsion and the jump of the canter at the same time as it stops the falling in or spinning around of the horse.

The outside leg, slightly behind the girth and supported by the outside rein, prevents the hindquarters from following the forehand in the same manner as for a volte. The weight of the rider rests increasingly on the inside seat bone but the upper body remains

vertical. The falling in of the rider's inside hip must at all costs be avoided, for this will have a disconcerting effect on the horse. The pirouette necessitates a horse that can remain in a certain frame and whose hindquarters can jump with ample impulsion under its own body. This is, however, only possible with light contact. Regardless of whether the horse performs a half, three-quarter or full pirouette, the aids are the same; it is only the number of canter jumps that varies. When the pirouette is completed, the rider must take more outside rein and at the same time drive forward with the inside leg. Both the seat bones must be weighed down and the hips pushed forward to rationalise the influence of the rider's lower back. The inside rein releases enough to allow the horse to adhere to the driving inside leg of the rider. The rhythm of the canter must neither be changed before, during or after the pirouette. The rider must be capable of ending the turn at any given time!

The pirouette cannot be taught on the long reins. However, it can be refined after it has been practised under the rider. As soon as the horse has understood the basic principles of the pirouette, the trainer can start to request the pirouette on the long reins. As before, the inside rein will lead the process of the turn, the outside rein offers support and the trainer moves in the direction of the movement of the pirouette in much the same way as with the beginning of the half pass. The outside rein frames the horse around the hindquarters and prevents the hindquarters from escaping. The trainer must at the same time bring the whip into play and lightly drive the horse sideways from the outside of the hindquarters. It is very important that the trainer does not tug the inside rein for this influences the flow of the movement and can cause a sudden interruption to the horse.

The trainer can also employ the shorter schooling whip, which has the advantage in that the trainer can tap a single hindleg when the need arises. It is naturally a good idea to be careful when tapping the hindlegs of the horse, you do not want the two hindlegs to jump at the same time. The canter beat must stay pure and must not be changed at all.

As said previously, the canter pirouette can be developed only under the rider and based on these grounds I would like to describe the most important exercises to achieve just that. At the Spanish Riding School, at first the canter pirouette is developed from the renvers. The renvers is the perfect technique to precede the pirouette, for the horse in renvers has the ideal frame and bend and is collected as well. The sequence canter-passade-renvers-pirouette is one of the classical exercises in the Spanish Riding School of Vienna. The horse canters on the long side of the arena, approximately in the middle of the arena the passade is initiated that will end roughly 5 metres from the track, the passade flows into the renvers at this point. Just before the corner the rider asks for a three-quarter pirouette and con-

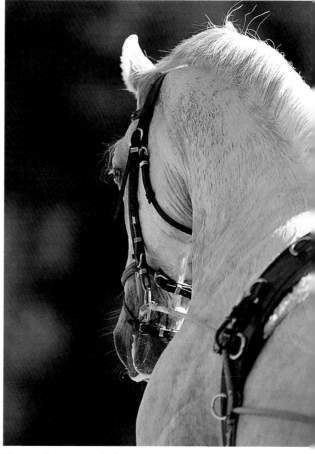

Eager anticipation on the long reins

tinues out of the pirouette into renvers once again. In the subsequent corner the next three-quarter pirouette is required. Once the horse starts to understand what is expected of him, a short walk or trot intermission follows and the lesson is then repeated. This must logically be repeated on both reins.

If the three-quarter pirouettes are too much to ask of the horse, it should only be expected to do half pirouettes. A further exercise at this point: the counter canter is ridden in a circle, at the open side of the circle a half pirouette is asked to the outside and the circle is repeated, this time on the correct canter lead. This exercise must also be repeated on both reins. The benefit of this exercise is easy to explain: the horse learns to enter the pirouette straight and to exit it straight, while in the pirouette learnt from the renvers, the horse will tend to become crooked before the execution of the pirouette. The disadvantage of the circle is that the rider does not have the same amount of control over the hindquarters as is the case in the renvers.

A further possibility for the development of the canter pirouette is the reduction of the circle, where the croup is slightly brought into the circle as if travers were required. The conclusion is a few pirouette jumps in the middle of the circle. Introduction and preliminary exercise is the volte ridden on the circle. The volte is at first required on the correct lead to the inside and later in the counter canter to the outside. Stronger aids on the outside will lead into the canter passade and then ultimately to the half pirouette to the outside. After these half pirouette jumps the canter strides should be lengthened somewhat to obtain a more powerful jump in the canter and to make up for lost impulsion. Soon afterwards the full pirouette can be attempted. To simplify the task a canter in renvers is executed on the circle. In order to keep the horse on his toes, the rider should alternate the aids between volte and pirouette so that the horse does not start to anticipate the next movement. Counter-acting a shoulder that falls in the plié canter (shoulder in at the canter) can be utilised, from which the pirouette can be introduced. Finally, the pirouette on a straight line is demanded and with that the classical objective is achieved.

FAULTS IN THE PIROUETTE, AND THEIR CORRECTION

The canter pirouette requires balance, impulsion, skill and most of all flexibility of the horse, all at the same time and because of this it is considered to be one of the most difficult manoeuvres in the art of classical riding. The occurrence of faults will therefore be correspondingly high. If one of the required abilities is absent or restricted the exercise will almost certainly fail. Owing to the numerous influencing factors and sources of failings, the trainer can gain insight into the status of the training and the attained "rideability" of the horse. The pirouette is therefore the measure of the quality of the training the horse has received.

The falling in shoulder:

This fault has already been described in the exercises. It is important that the horse waits for the aids and pays an adequate amount of attention to the inside leg, for this reason we alternate between the pirouette and the volte. The pirouette can furthermore be expected from the shoulder in as well. The introduction of the pirouette from the walk can also be a solution. The horse is asked for a pirouette in the walk and from this the canter pirouette is then required. This is an exceptionally beneficial technique for highly strung horses.

Carrying the pirouette too far:

This is mainly a rider problem when the rider cannot end the pirouette at a specific point. The pirouette can be interrupted by a halt or walk transition. In both cases the horse should continue straight on in walk and repeats the canter pirouette once more. The second possibility is to ride the pirouette from the canter half pass and to end it with a canter half pass.

Croup falling out at the beginning of the pirouette:

The pirouette becomes more like a volte with this fault. As with the falling in of the shoulder, the horse will choose to ignore the aids and attempt to break away from the collection. This fault can be rectified when the trainer develops the pirouette from the renvers as described earlier. With the renvers the trainer has much more control over the croup of the horse.

Running out of steam:

Although the horse turns on the spot, he almost discontinues the canter – he runs out of steam. The root of this problem can be eradicated by making the pirouette bigger. In a perfect world the horse canters the pirouette almost on one spot roughly the size of a dinner plate. For the correction of this fault the size of the pirouette must be increased and the trainer must expect many half pirouettes as opposed to full

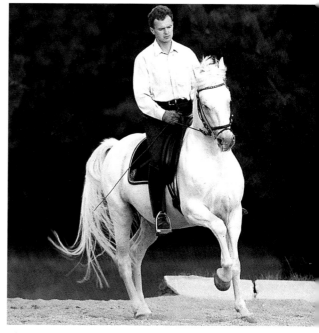

The canter pirouette is the measure of "rideability".

pirouettes at first. Once the trainer is satisfied that the horse can maintain the canter, the full pirouette can be demanded again.

Jumping back in the pirouette:

The influence of the rider's hand is too strong. In most cases a softer, more giving hand will already be a solution to the problem. If this is not the case, the same modification as was the basis for curing "running out of steam" can be applied. If the backwards tendency goes together with the fast swinging round of the forehand, the same correction used in the falling in shoulders can be brought into play. The most important factor in all the above-mentioned faults, is that the impulsion must be kept going and the horse must maintain the forward tendency at all times.

In the same way as the capriole and levade can be cultivated from the piaffe, different elements of the airs above the ground can be acquired from the terre à terre, for example the courbette and mézair. In exactly the same way as the piaffe, the terre à terre is also achieved from the unhurried shortening of the gait. The canter is gently, without robbing the horse's impulsion, shortened until the jumps turn out to be more elevated with little forward movement. In the beginning it is wise to require only a few such short canter jumps. In the course of time the trainer can demand increasingly shortened canter strides until the horse canters on the spot. It is important to allow the horse to relax with increased impulsion after the powerful phase of shortening – I normally allow the horse to canter briskly in an extensive circle. This lesson can be developed under the rider at the same time. The seat of the rider is extremely significant at this point, the horse must always be in front of the rider, in other words the driving aids must predominate over the restraining hand!

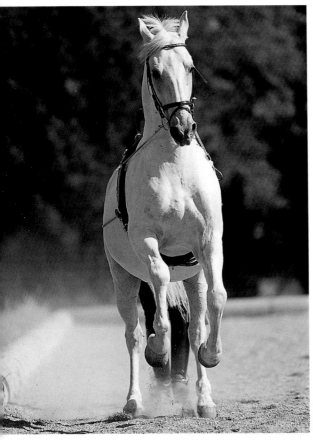

A high-quality terre à terre develops from a dynamic canter

THE TERRE À TERRE

When the horse is capable of executing full halt transitions from the canter, the next stage is another gait in the high school training. This has long been forgotten in the competitive sport we know today: the canter at a standstill, also known as the terre à terre. The terre à terre has a great gymnastic value as well as practical application.

FLYING CHANGE

The flying change is a change of the canter lead in the moment of suspension without interruption from the halt, walk or trot transition. The old masters insisted that the horse must not be expected to perform the flying change until it is strong enough and possesses sufficient suppleness. This expectation is justifiable because the change is required in the moment of suspension and is only possible when the hindquarters are powerful enough to achieve an adequate amount of lift for this to happen. Even more important is that the horse must be in perfect balance. The following basic demands can therefore be made for the flying change:

> *The flying change should only be demanded once the horse is capable of moving forward with lively, regular and unchanging canter strides.*

A thorough preparation is compulsory when the flying change is to be learned. This can be done under the rider as well as on the long reins. The actual performance of the flying change on the long reins is to be advised against if the trainer is not an absolute master of the art of long reining. Once the preparation for the flying change has been done on the long reins as well as under the rider, the best way to advance is to execute the flying change under the rider first. Once the change is well established under the rider, it can also be performed on the long reins or the shortened long reins as will be described later.

A vastly important point to remember in the flying change is that the horse must "jump through", meaning that the change must be done with the hindlegs as well as the front legs at the same time. It is good practice to have an experienced rider to

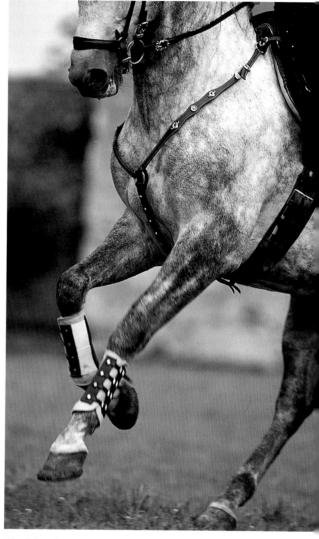

The flying change is required only once the horse is capable of elevated canter strides

keep an eye on the work for the flying change from the ground, just to relate to the trainer if the horse is executing the change correctly or in two phases! The change in two phases is when the forelegs change first and then the hindlegs change in the next canter stride. If the change is and possibly even the canter pirouette. A horse capable of this is in general well equipped to perform the flying change and the trainer can without delay continue to the special preparations.

The special preparations lie in making the horse sensitive to the new canter aids. The aids for the flying change are exactly the same as for the simple change; the only difference being the horse does not perform the half-halt into the trot transition. The horse should be able to change only from the aids coming from the legs, reins and the corresponding, invisible weight shift. There are often varieties of contortions to be seen in the arena when riders attempt the flying change; these are not only unnecessary, but also cumbersome for the horse. If the flying change is taught with quiet and correct aids there will be no irreparable faults or problems that require long-term solutions. The next exercise is an excellent preparatory technique on long reins for the flying change: collected canter – trot transition – counter canter – trot transition – canter and so on. The distances between right and left canter become shorter until the horse scarcely shows any steps in trot. Once the horse is this far, the trot transitions can be replaced with walk transitions, right canter – walk transition – left canter – walk transition. The distances between the canters must also be shortened until the horse almost has only one walk stride left. This is almost a flying change, albeit without the moment of sus-

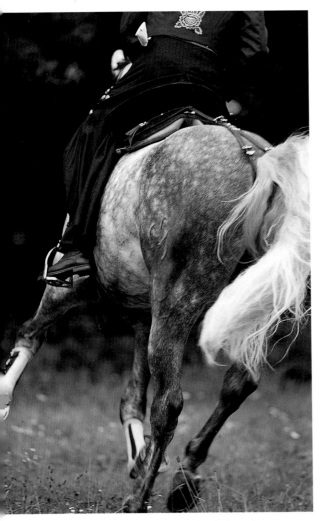

It is enormously important that the horse jumps through right from the start of the flying change

the other way around, in other words the horse changes with the hindlegs first and then changes the forelegs, it is not such a grave fault, for the horse will in a short time become skilled enough to accomplish the change correctly. By this stage of training, the horse is proficient in the lateral gaits as well as the piaffe and terre à terre pension. The same lesson must be applied under the rider as well. The rider will find the horse wishes suddenly to change by himself. Extensive praise should then be given and the lesson brought to an end. In my experience it is better to teach the flying change on the one leg first and later to the other leg and only once the horse is competent on both sides to combine the two.

There are many more techniques to produce the flying change itself. A few of those deserve a mention in passing: canter – half a circle from the corner – half pass back to the track and on the track the flying change into the correct lead. Another possibility is the counter canter on the long side of the arena in renvers and then flying change into the correct lead. The flying change can also be attempted from the plié canter. As previously described, the plié-canter is a canter in a shoulder in. The change from the shoulder in has the advantage that the hindquarters are under control to the greatest possible extent due to the amount of collection of the lateral gait. Although the flying change can be taught from the lateral movements, the goal should still be to perform the change on the straight line. The horse should be performing the flying change on straight lines at the right time. One possibility is to position the horse straight just before the aids are given for the flying change; this is a clever way to produce a changeover phase. Yet another variation is the flying

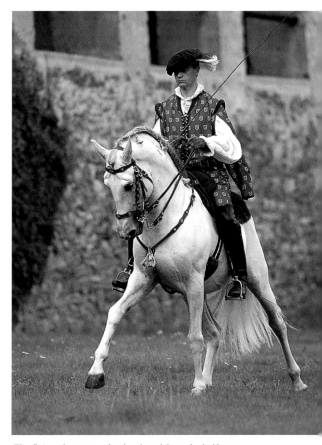

The flying change can be developed from the half pass at the canter

change from the halt; this is especially beneficial for nervous and flighty horses. The trainer will now place a transition into halt between the left and right canter, which becomes so short that the horse changes with a second or two to spare. If the rider is skilled enough, the horse can be persuaded to perform a flying change through the right amount of driving aids. The flying change can also be developed from the lengthened or medium canter, for the canter is stretched out across the diagonal and with the shortening to the collected canter the flying change can be requested. The advantage of this is obvious, for it will promote the impulsion and forward drive the flying change requires. Not all the exercises can be used to the same effect on different horses. Thus it can happen that an exercise is perfectly suitable today and have absolutely no value tomorrow and another exercise has to be substituted for it. This does not, however, mean that the old exercise cannot be used again the day after. The thinking rider is always challenged in the training, but especially so in the flying change. Mindless riding according to instructions, without thinking about the outcome or even the reason for the lessons, will create mindless horses. It is also a natural feature that the rider should praise the horse after it has achieved success, even if it is really small! Punishment in the flying change especially has no rationale, for this is the one time where practice makes perfect. This extends to the horse that offers the flying change without being called upon, never punish him for it. If the trainer often changes the specific place where the aids are given for the flying change, the horse will start to wait for the command. There are, of course, many more ways to develop the flying change; the trainer's own creativity should also be drawn out! Teaching the horse a series of changes, such as four, three, two and single changes should be left to professional trainers. There are too few riders that have enough ability to teach their horses this difficult lesson.

FAULTS IN THE FLYING CHANGE, AND THEIR CORRECTION

Correction of faults in the flying change should only be attempted under the rider, for the influence on the long reins is too limited.

Jumping in two phases:

This is the one fault that is most often found in the flying change and is the result of too little collection. This could be because the preconditions were not sufficient, due to the rider's inability, or simply because the horse is not yet at the right stage of his training to be able to do this. In any of the above-mentioned situations the rider is to blame. The problem now is to build enough power in the horse and to put him in balance or if that is already the state of affairs, to perform the special exercises as correction. These are the flying change from the lateral gaits or from the quarter or half pirouette, for the horse already needs to be in collection for all of these exercises.

The horse changes crooked:

This is when the change is crooked to one side, for it should be perfectly straight. Most of the time the fault lies in the excessive application of the aids and the weight change of the rider. Once the cause is removed, the flying change must be demanded in a higher tempo, for example the medium canter. The difference should be noted within a reasonable short time.

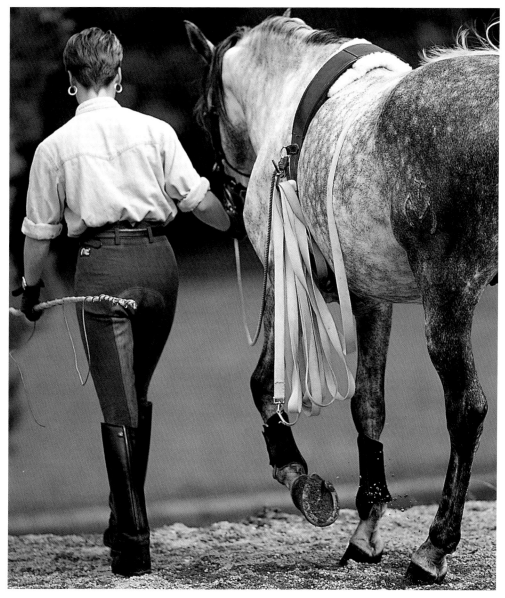

Returning to the stable satisfied

Arresting the flying change:

The horse shortens the last stride before the change so much that he almost stops. The best remedy for this is to ask for the change from a medium canter, without collecting the horse too much, for that may exacerbate the problem. The seat of the rider must in this situation also be scrutinised, for this fault can easily develop when the rider's body goes in front of the vertical.

Running after the flying change:

The main cause for this is overzealous application of the aids or the horse's fear of too strong a collection. To solve the second part of the problem the horse should be strengthened in order to lose the fear of collection. The first problem is resolved with finer and subtler application of the aids.

If both of these fail, the change should be requested with the interruption of a halt, as has been described already. The horse will soon break the habit and perform the flying change correctly.

Quick change:

The horse does not change with an elevated and forward jump, but quickly changes between two canter strides. This fault develops when the horse is not yet powerful enough to perform the flying change and therefore the moment of suspension is too short to make for an impressive and beautiful change. The horse should in such a situation be given more time to strengthen the hindquarters before attempting the flying change again.

In general the consensus, as far as the faults in the flying change are concerned, is:

If the horse lacks the strength in the hindquarters to perform a high enough jump, the moment of suspension is not long enough to coordinate the legs in the flying change. Lack of strength in the hindquarters is therefore a big source of problems.

SUMMARY OF THE WORK
ON THE LONG REINS

· *Commencing with collection:*
  short turns and turn on the haunches,
  shoulder in and simple changes, halt
  transitions from all three gaits;
  getting used to the double bridle with
  the rider up.
· *Medium collection: start of the piaffe,*
  travers, half pass, renvers.
· *Full collection: pirouettes, flying change,*
  passage, series of changes, commencing the refinement of the work in hand.

Training
in Hand according
to the Iberian School

Training in hand according to the Iberian school is very specialised and only really effective when the horse has been prepared with the preceding work on the long reins. The exception is in sideways overstepping in hand, with which the lateral gaits can be complemented on the long reins. This work can be used right from the start on the young Iberian horses and other horses that are extremely sensitive and rather temperamental in their behaviour, this kind of work was devised for these types of horses in the first place. There are also those horses on which this training in hand using the Iberian methods is not possible, as is often the situation with thoroughbred horses. The advantages of the Iberian training in hand are that less equipment is required, no

helper is needed and there is always the possibility of relaxing the horse in between exercises. This training focuses in particular on the lateral gaits, the piaffe, the passage and the Spanish walk, the Spanish trot and the levade.

The question arises: Why? All of the above have already been taught on the long reins. The answer is as follows: every lesson that the horse has already learnt on the long reins will be refined and perfected in the step by step technique of this training in hand. The horse must learn to develop into a round outline and move forward in perfect balance.

Granted, all lessons that are possible on the long reins can be worked at in the Iberian manner, but it can only be achieved with horses that are sensitive enough.

throws the croup up. In addition, due to the close proximity of the trainer to the horse and the intensive work, it is easy for the trainer to annoy or scare the horse.

EQUIPMENT

Unlike many of the other techniques, there is almost no need for any special equipment in this kind of training. The only piece of equipment that the trainer should attach any importance to is the whip to touch the horse with. I personally prefer natural rods of beech wood, which can be cut to the exact length you want, or the whips of quince wood used (and only found) in Portugal. The reason for my almost old-fashioned partiality to these whips lies in the fact that the whips that can be bought nowadays seldom have the action that I need. When speaking of the correct action of a whip, I refer to its elasticity in relation to its length. The ultimate whip will therefore be quite stiff in the first two thirds and relatively elastic in the last third. When the whip is soft and elastic through the whole length, the aid will not be presented at the precise moment, but too late. If the whip is too rigid throughout its length, there will be little effect and the trainer's hand will tire rapidly. If a suitable whip, which fulfils all criteria, is found in a specialist shop, there is nothing to prevent one from buying it.

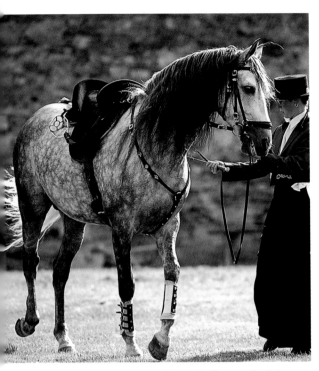

When training according to the Iberian school the trainer is close to the horse. In this picture the shoulder in left is seen.

On the basis of my own experience I have found that the measures described here have proven to be the best techniques to train the horse. They have also brought the best quality results while not over exerting the horse.

The trainer is very close to the horse in the Iberian technique and the aids can therefore become exceptionally refined, but on the other hand the bigger picture can easily be lost because of this proximity. For example, the trainer can become focused on the mobilisation of the hindquarters of the horse in the piaffe and forget to observe whether the forehand is in the correct position or fail to notice that the horse only

The length of the whip depends on the size of the horse and the trainer and must be chosen individually. Gloves are, as always in work in hand, a definite requirement.

PRECONDITIONS AND FIRST TRAINING STEPS

Training in hand, as implemented on the Iberian peninsula, is normally required before the daily ridden work, to warm up the horse without the rider and to prepare him for the work under saddle. In particular, it is easier when training is first started with the horse, to perform the exercises with the rider dismounted. The trainer will mostly stand on the inside of the horse and begin the work on the left side of the horse. The horse wears a normal saddle and bridle. The left hand of the trainer holds the left rein in close proximity to the snaffle bit, the right hand holds the right rein that goes over the neck just in front of the withers. The whip is also held in the right hand of the trainer, as one would hold a fencing foil, ready to touch the horse on the rump, flank, croup or legs.

The training of the horse according to the Iberian school is, as you would expect, also possible in a double bridle and is practised this way on the Iberian peninsula. The reins are held in the 2:2 and the Fillis way, as has been described. If only a curb

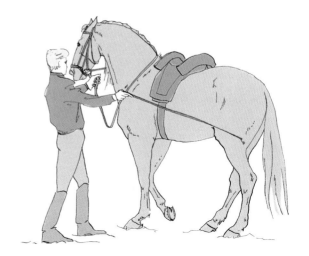

Correct method of holding the reins and whip when training according to the Iberian school

bit is used, which is only possible without damage with highly schooled horses, the reins are held correspondingly with the softness used for the snaffle bit. Another option, especially in the more elevated work of the piaffe, passage or levade, is to keep both reins in one hand as in the ridden work, over the withers of the horse. This application of the reins will leave the other hand of the trainer free to touch the horse on any or all of the points needed.

The work in hand should commence from the halt. The horse is stroked all over its body with the whip.

The trainer shows the horse the whip, then strokes it over the horse on the neck, back, croup, legs and abdomen, to reassure and comfort the horse. Only once the horse stays calm when touched all over his body with the whip, does the trainer commence the actual work. The first exercise, to get the horse used to the new manner of working, is the halt transition from the walk. The request for the walk follows a vocal demand and the touching of the horse on the ribs where the legs of the rider would normally be. This is repeated on both reins until the horse moves forward in a relaxed and free walk. In this period the trainer should develop a feeling for the strength with which the whip aids need to be applied, but at the same time he must acquire a feeling for the rein aids. The trainer can get the horse on the bit with light vibration on the reins. As soon as the horse comes on the bit and moves in the carriage the trainer expects from him, the hand must give and become softer. At this stage the horse will begin to chew the bit. This exercise is repeated on both reins until the horse flexes in his poll and does not lean on the hand of the trainer.

The trainer, who has been walking at the head of the horse till now, must move rearwards to approximately next to the horse's shoulder. This is the correct position to work with the horse. The position of the trainer has a big influence on the horse, the further to the rear of the horse, the more driving the position, the further to the front of the horse, the greater the constraining effect. The transition into the halt is achieved through a half-halt on the outside rein, the inside rein is applied only if the horse does not react. The half-halt is not much more than merely a light vibration with the hand; always remember, it takes two to pull! The purpose of this work is, as with the training on the lunge and long reins, to prepare a highly sensitive horse with aids as light as possible. Only when the horse manages the halt from the walk without difficulty can the halt from the trot be attempted. Once these exercises are successful, the horse is required to rein back and to move straight into trot again from three of four steps in the rein back. When the horse accepts all these lessons willingly, the trainer can expect the same lessons the horse has learnt on the long reins in order to refine them. Do not forget to praise the horse in this work!

STEPPING LATERALLY UNDER THE BODY

Stepping laterally under the body around the forehand is the first lesson of the Iberian training and teaches the horse the driving aids to the side. The horse is asked to come in an outline in the middle of the arena, far away from the wall. The whip is used to touch the horse on its barrel at the height of the stifle joint and care must be taken that the horse does not step forward too far.

When the horse reacts on the aids with the desired sideways step, the whip and

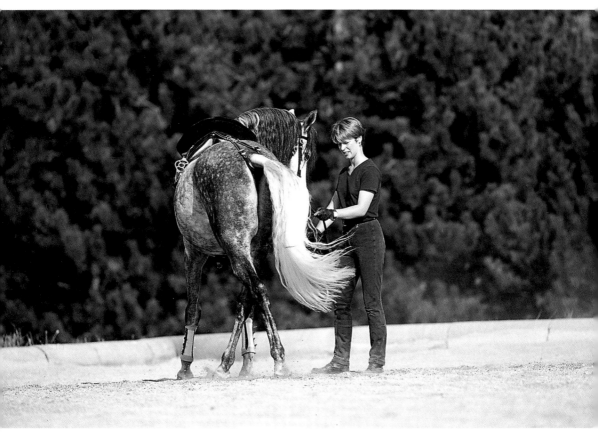

Stepping laterally under the body

LATERAL WORK

hand are dropped and the horse praised. If no reaction is shown, the whip aid should be increased and an extra aid in the form of a click from the trainer's tongue given. This exercise is done on both reins; only a few steps are demanded in order not to irritate the horse. Once the horse is capable of this on both reins in the walk, the trainer asks for it in the trot as well.

By this time the horse is used to this work and the moment has arrived where further lateral movements can be added reminiscent of the ones already cultivated under the rider as well as on the long reins. The trainer starts with the easiest lesson of the lateral gaits, the shoulder in, where the trainer moves next to the inside shoulder of the horse.

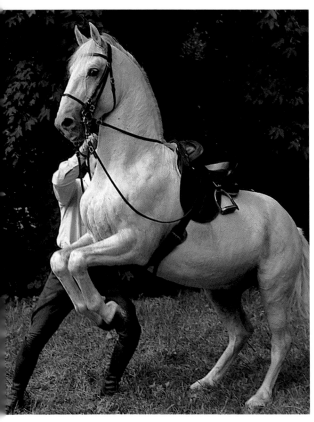

Levade in hand in the Iberian manner

slightly in. Two or three steps of shoulder in are requested, if the horse pushes to the inside of the arena, the inside hand vibrates in an upward movement to work in opposition to the inside push of the horse. The whip taps the barrel lightly or if the horse is too sensitive, just lies against the side of the horse. The exercise of the shoulder in is also started in the walk and practised on both reins until the horse feels comfortable performing it along the side of the arena without problems. The shoulder in must every now and again be interrupted by a halt transition and the horse must be able to stand completely still and relaxed. Now the horse can be asked for a few strides in trot. The trot commences from the shoulder in on the walk. The transition into trot is made without straightening the horse, and after a few strides the horse is half-halted into the walk, only to trot again after some walk strides. This naturally is repeated a couple of times on both the left and the right rein.

After the work in hand, the same sequence is repeated under saddle and the walk transition can be replaced with transitions into halt, which makes the exercise more demanding. In both situations, under the rider as well as in hand, the outside rein and the driving inside aids are of great importance. Repetition of this lesson not only demonstrates the accuracy of the aids, but will also correct the horse if it does not accept the outside rein or inside leg (inside whip), or only acknowledges it faintly.

Once again, the position of the trainer is extremely important: to the front of the horse it will have a restraining effect, further to the rear it will have a driving influence. The degree to which the trainer's position has to be changed will depend greatly on the horse; the trainer must simply try various positions to discover which suits the horse best. For a start the trainer must get the horse in an outline next to the wall of the arena, the head of the horse

Once the horse can effortlessly perform these lessons, the trainer moves on to the next exercise: shoulder in at the start of the long side of the arena, diagonal change in shoulder in to about the midline. There the horse is turned around the hocks, still in the shoulder in, and returned to the track and continued along the long side of the arena in counter shoulder in. Both corners will be executed in counter shoulder in. When the horse arrives on the next long side of the arena, the trainer must carefully change the horse over into the shoulder in on the other rein and proceed across the diagonal in half pass.

A further option to initiate the half pass in hand is to give the aids from a half volte or from the midline. At first the half pass is asked on the rein that is easier for the horse. If this is the left hand, the trainer leads the horse against the wall on the right rein, he walks on the inside of the horse, leads it from the middle, changes the bend to the left and drives it carefully but positively sideways. Once this exercise can successfully be completed, the trainer will demand travers against the long side of the arena as well as renvers. There are two approaches to teach renvers in hand. In the first place: in the diagonal from the half pass, the croup of the horse is taken over further in the changeover to the long side of the arena, the shoulder is held and the horse goes into renvers. In the second place the renvers is developed from the shoulder in at the walk, where the trainer

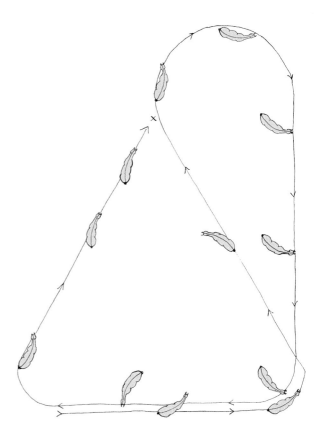

Lateral work in the Iberian method: shoulder in turn on the haunches – counter shoulder in and transition to the half pass

carefully bends the horse in the other direction, the direction of the movement. Later the trainer can also request volte in renvers and ask for the circle to be decreased and increased in renvers.

Lateral work should only be requested once both the trainer and horse are confident in the work in hand and exercises like the lateral stepping under the body and the shoulder in cause no more difficulty.

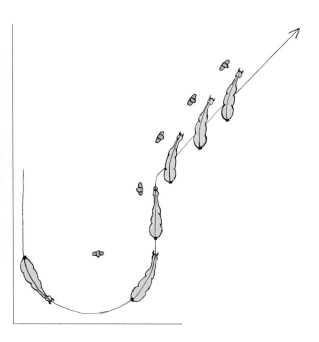

Commencing the half pass from the midline

The advantage of training according to the Iberian school is that the trainer can correct and control the bend and outline of the horse to a greater degree. The trainer should take great care not to overbend the horse for this fault is even graver than too little bend. To prevent this fault from occurring, the trainer takes the horse forward with more tempo and does not bend the horse quite as much. The impulsion and forward movement of the gait is also very important in this situation. Many horses will lose momentum, especially in renvers; this can be avoided if the trainer goes nearer the middle of the arena.

I should now like to repeat some of the most important basics of the lateral work in hand: because the reins are simultaneously brought into play, the inside rein is the one that forms the bend. The trainer is positioned between the horse and the wall of the arena in the travers and the half pass, which is on the opposite side of the bend. In shoulder in and renvers the reverse is true, the trainer is on the inside of the horse, which is between the trainer and the wall of the arena.

In the course of the work on the lateral gaits, the rein back in hand must also be introduced. In order to achieve this the horse is halted next to the side of the arena with the trainer at the shoulder of the horse. With the legs slightly spread the trainer must lean the upper body backwards towards the horse's croup and shift the body weight onto the leg that is more to the rear. The connection to the horse's mouth stays elastic throughout and with light tension and pull on the reins, the trainer asks the horse to step back one or two strides. When this is successful, the hand gives immediately and the horse is praised extensively. Then the reins are taken up and the lesson is repeated once more. Later on in the training extra strides are expected until the amount of steps called for are achieved (about one horse's length).

At this point the "Schaukel" or "swing" can additionally be requested. This is three or four steps of rein back followed , without halting, by three or four steps forwards in walk, and again, without halting, three or four steps of rein back. A short trot can also be expected within this lesson and additional lessons can be reiterated.

"GOAT ON THE MOUNTAIN TOP"

The next exercise might be unfamiliar to a number of readers; it is one that extends back to the teachings of Baucher. He developed the exercise for horses that are frightened when their front and hind legs come into close proximity to each other. It is also valuable for horses with long backs that tend to let their legs trail. Horses that naturally have their forelegs more under their bodies are not taught this, for it will be counter-productive. This lesson has the appropriate name of "mêtre l'isard sur un pic" (goat on the mountain top) and is a means to an end. This lesson helps horses that feel over anxious when collected.

The trainer halts the horse on the track and taps one canon bone with the whip until the horse places it more underneath its body. The same is then required from the other leg. Do not ask too much at the beginning. The horse receives a titbit as reward, always and only in the low stretched position. The horse may not step forward unless asked to do so. After a while, with the necessary practice, the

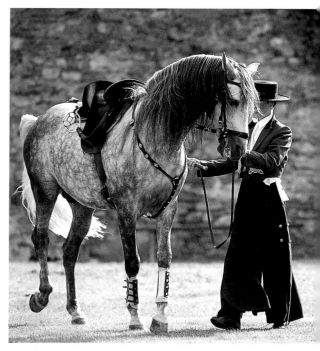

Left shoulder in: Julepe and Claudia Dietz

horse will be able to move his hindlegs about 20 centimetres forward towards the front legs. When the horse is capable of performing this without a problem, it is demanded under the rider as well. At the same time as the rider prevents the horse from stepping forward, the trainer taps the legs of the horse with the whip until they move under the body of the horse. Once this is also a success, the trainer can ask the horse (without the rider) to frame

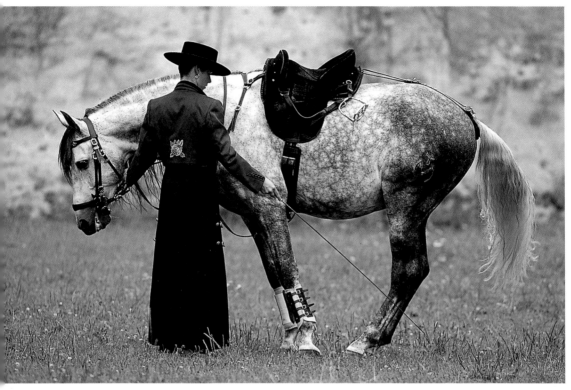

"Goat on the mountain top": the low head carriage is important for it stretches the whole topline

himself and put more weight on the hindquarters. Now the trainer can ask a few piaffe steps, which have already been practised on the long reins, with the aid of the clicking tongue and galvanising tapping of the whip.

This exercise will also be valuable in the work between the pillars at a later point in time. I have often taught this lesson as a preliminary exercise for the piaffe in the long reins. Combinations of different pos-

sibilities in the training are always workable, it all depends on the ability and natural talent of the individual horse.

PIAFFE

The piaffe is developed exactly as with the long reins, through the systematic shortening of the trot stride. This is established on the track where the trainer taps the horse on the rump, flank or hindquarters while at the same time preventing the horse from going forward with the hand.

Because the trainer stands so close to the horse, it is always possible to tap the horse more precisely than in the work on the long reins. In this work it may be necessary to plait the horse's tail in a knot and put it in a tail fastener to keep the legs of the horse free and allowing the whip to be used without hindrance. In the chapter "Training in hand according to the Viennese school", the reactions will be discussed when the horse is tapped on specific points. Not all positions are easily reached with the whip in the Iberian way for the trainer also has to hold the reins.

In order to reach a highly collected piaffe, the horse can be requested to piaffe from the rein back, or as on the long reins, from the lateral movement. The piaffe can also be developed from the shoulder in. The shoulder in as a lesson and correction is of superior value in the art of riding and can almost be seen as a "cure all". It is therefore not surprising that it can be utilised in a profitable way in the piaffe work. The transition from the shoulder in to the piaffe will mostly be used when the horse hurries and with a horse that is more temperamental. Once again, the shoulder in is started on the side that is easy for the horse. The trainer must now tap the horse with such galvanising accuracy that the horse will increase the frequency of its steps and progress into a diagonal footfall. With the first piaffe-like steps the trainer

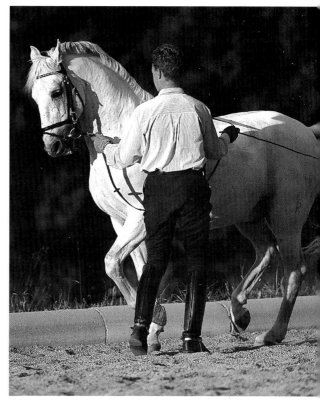

Maestoso Ancona in the piaffe in hand.

must relax the hand and praise the horse, and soon after repeat the lesson a few times on both reins. The influence of the trainer should as always be delicate and inviting, not sharp and forceful. He must attempt to transfer his energy to the horse without making it nervous or anxious. Once the piaffe is favourably performed, the passage can also be requested in the Iberian manner.

DEVELOPMENT OF THE PASSAGE FROM THE PIAFFE

The ideal way to develop the passage is from the piaffe, as has already been discussed and the trainer stands on the inside of the horse for this exercise. The trainer allows the horse, without losing the rhythmical tapping, to step more forwards, similar to the shortened or collected trot. If the horse feels restricted or the trainer gets the feeling that he cannot move on, the tempo can be increased but the trainer must always take great care to stay somewhat in front of the horse's shoulder to prevent the horse from running away. After a short episode in which the horse actually shows some cadenced passage steps, the work is paused and the horse praised. This is then repeated on the other rein; only a few steps are expected for the horse must not be overtaxed. Certain horses react better to the tapping of the front end (corresponding points can be found on p.138). Passage in hand using the Iberian technique is a little more difficult to teach the horse, I usually start the passage on the long reins and only use the Iberian technique to refine the passage.

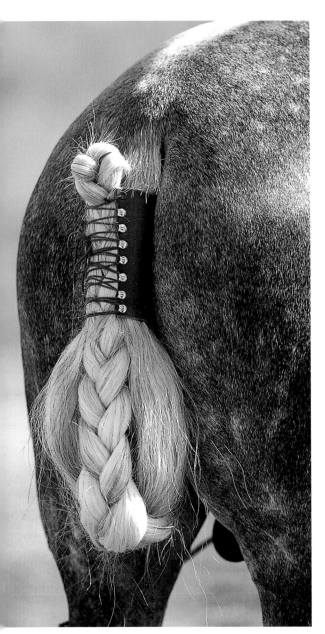

The tail in a plait in a tail fastener

THE SPANISH WALK

The alternate lifting of the front legs to the horizontal while keeping the walk sequence is denoted the Spanish walk.

This is often mistaken for the Spanish step, which is nothing other than an old word for the passage. The preliminary exercises for the Spanish walk demands some patience from the trainer! The trainer starts the horse on a free line and stands on the left side of the horse, takes both reins in one hand, either directly next to the horse's mouth or somewhat shortened at the horse's withers, and then taps the front leg of the horse on different points to find out where the horse shows the most reaction. Several horses will respond apathetically to this experiment at first, either by not reacting at all or by evading sideways or backwards. If the evasion is to the side, the trainer positions the horse on the track, for the evasion to the back the trainer must tap the horse lightly on the hindquarters to counteract this. If this still does not help, the horse is positioned in a corner to be framed with another wall. The trainer should never become impatient with the horse, for it is only with patience, not force, that this can be achieved.

A small digression in horse psychology will explain a little: the Spanish walk is not an unnatural tutorial. Stallions that challenge each other to play or fight will often strike with the foreleg in this manner, sometimes even repeatedly. This can be evoked when the horse is in a playful, boisterous or aggressive mood. The trainer must therefore be absolutely meticulous to pay attention never to allow the horse to be frightened when expecting this lesson, for

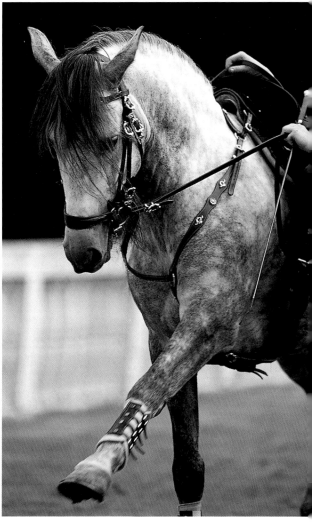

The Spanish walk: the whip serves only as support, the horse reacts to the hand aids to raise the prevailing leg

the horse may never perform this in a state of anxiety.

The trainer can also take advantage of the psychology behind the Spanish walk, for this is the natural way to deflate

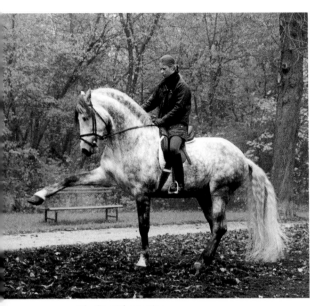

The Spanish greeting

way the trainer wants it to be stretched, it often helps to use a toothpick and prick the horse under the forearm from behind while a helper taps the designated position with the whip. The tapping of the whip should be inviting and not too intense. The feeling of the whip should be similar to an annoying fly that will most certainly result in the horse stamping its feet.

If the horse keeps his leg in the air for some time, this is the Spanish greeting. This lesson can be triggered from the saddle as well when the rider touches the horse's shoulder from above and in that way trigger the same reaction as in hand.

Once the horse can accomplish this, the trainer can start to expect the lifting of the leg in the walk. The trainer has the horse on the track, stands on the inside and requests a walk. From this intense walk the trainer can then ask, with the aid of the whip, that the horse lifts his forelegs in the movement. If this is successful, without losing any of the forward travel, the trainer repeats the same lesson on the other rein as well. Once the horse is capable of performing this with both legs, the trainer can start to demand the lifting of alternated legs, but always with two walk steps between: for example – lift left – two walk strides – lift right – two walk strides and so forth. This exercise is called the "Polka". With some horses it is often better to ask for only one leg to be lifted at first. Later on, when the exercise is established, the other leg can be asked to lift in the walk,

aggression or anger, that can be easily built up during training, and the Spanish walk presents an outlet for that pent-up energy. A second extremely positive training benifitof the Spanish walk is the enormous freedom at the shoulder the horse develops in this lesson and that is worth its weight in gold when it comes to the piaffe and passage.

Now to return to the exercise before us: when the horse shows any reaction, for example by pawing, stamping or any kind of lifting of the leg (and that can take a while), it is praised extensively, and given a titbit as a reward. Then, of course, the whole exercise is repeated on the other side. This exercise is performed until the horse lifts or even stretches the prevailing leg when it is tapped lightly. If, however, the horse does not stretch his leg in the and the two exercises are then combined into the alternating lift of the legs in the polka.

Once the training has progressed this far, the Spanish walk is almost achieved: the trainer asks for only a few strides with the alternate lifting of the legs at each stride. Keep the sequence very short so the horse does not lose the rhythm of the walk. It is also important to keep an eye on the horse's placement of the hindlegs and make sure that he steps under his body properly, for the better the step under, the better the lift in the forehand.

The horse is now taught under the rider to lift the appropriate leg when he lifts the rein on the same side. In the Spanish walk, in much the same manner as in the normal walk, the rider must still drive the horse forward in the same rhythm. At first, this is easier when the rider adds the tapping aid of the whip on the shoulder of the horse to complement the rein aid.

One will often see how a rider accomplishes the Spanish walk by stretching his own leg forward towards the horse's shoulder and at the same time shifting his body weight to the opposite side. I personally am not partial to this way of doing things, for it will usually cause the horse to sway from one side to the other in a rather drunken fashion - not exactly an aesthetic picture. For future work, this way will not help the Spanish trot, for it is almost impossible for the rider to lift his leg in alternate rhythm from the side of the horse and push it to the

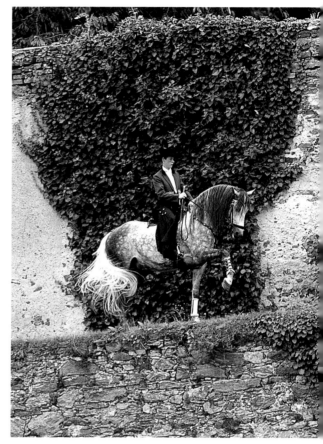

Claudia Dietz in the Spanish walk on Julepe

shoulder of the horse. If the rider is capable of such gymnastics on horseback he is definitely an exceptional talent!

The rider must always take care that the horse does not stumble and fall. The complete and accurate learning of the Spanish walk will take up to one year to accomplish. The horse should then be capable of performing the Spanish walk at any time and any place for at least 60 metres in the correct sequence of footfalls.

will promote the energetic lift of the foreleg. This problem will disappear soon enough, provided that the rider has put a stop to the exaggerated shift in his own body weight and sits quietly and straight on the centre of gravity of the horse.

The hindquarters stay behind:

In this situation the trainer demands too many steps – less is always more! The correction for this is also the tapping of the hindlegs by a helper.

The horse lifts the front legs insufficiently:

This is a situation where the horse must either be given time to develop his own ability with practice into the higher lift demanded, or the trainer must put more pressure on the horse and demand more intensely to obtain the desired reaction.

SPANISH WALK IN THE REIN BACK

Once the horse remains calm and controlled in the Spanish walk, the trainer can ask that the horse performs this in the rein back as well.

The horse lifts alternate front legs, but when the front legs are placed on the ground, the horse steps back in the correct footfall, namely in diagonal pairs. The Spanish walk in the rein back is frequently less problematic for the horse to perform. The trainer takes the horse to the track again and stands on the inside of the horse once more, this time slightly

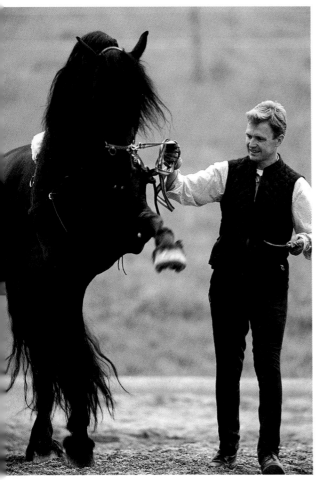

The Spanish walk can later be demanded in the Viennese way

FAULTS IN THE SPANISH WALK, AND THEIR CORRECTION

Swaying in the Spanish walk:

Many horses are prone to this kind of movement, although it is mostly a rider fault as has been described. The correction is for a helper to drive the horse forward in the walk with the aid of a whip on the hindleg, this more at the front of the horse's shoulder, bringing into play the restraining position. The trainer now requests a rein back – halt – lifting of the inside front leg – rein back – halt – lifting of the inside front leg.

The trainer continues to ask the horse to lift first the one leg and then the other. With patience on the part of the trainer, the horse will soon learn to lift his legs alternately and step back at the same time. The trainer must not ignore the forward tendency of the horse and therefore should keep this lesson in the rein back relatively short.

DEVELOPING THE PASSAGE FROM THE SPANISH WALK

If the horse is accomplished in performing the Spanish walk at signals from the whip, the basis is in place for developing of the passage from the Spanish walk. The horse is asked to trot from the Spanish walk, where he steps under himself correctly, in a collected manner and the trainer taps the horse with the whip on the normal positions as is the case with the Spanish trot itself. The work is interrupted and the horse praised the minute he shows some cadenced and elevated steps. The trainer continues in this way for days, weeks or even months until the horse can perform many more steps for longer stretches at a time.

Once again it is an advantage to teach this in hand first. The choice of developing the passage in this way according to the

Iberian technique in hand or on the long reins is still subject to the trainer's own judgement and preference. In the meantime, it is useful to have a helper who can drive the horse with the whip on the hindlegs to prevent them from staying behind the movement.

There are disadvantages of teaching the passage from the Spanish walk: there is frequently a danger of confusing the Spanish walk and the passage with each other, for the horse often cannot understand the difference between the two gaits. Apart from that, the horse is in better collection when the passage is developed from the piaffe. For this reason I prefer teaching the passage from the piaffe. There is another problem when the horse is taught the passage from the Spanish walk; many horses use the rein as support and overbend in the process of trying to lean on the bit. This method of teaching the horse the passage must therefore only be used in specific situations on individual horses.

PIROUETTE ON THREE LEGS

The pirouette on three legs is when the horse keeps one leg lifted as in the Spanish greeting and then performs a turn on the forehand.

This is an artificial lesson that I would, all the same, like to describe, for it does not cause any harm when performed occasionally, appears delightful and demands a high degree of obedience from the horse.

In the pirouette to the left the horse must stay put with his right leg on the ground while the left leg is lifted as high as possible. The position is, of course, reversed for the pirouette to the right. If the horse has already learnt the Spanish walk or the Spanish greeting, it is simply a question of patience and practice.

The horse stands in the middle of the arena; the trainer stands on the horse's left, next to the rump, and asks through the tapping of the whip on the right shoulder, breast or leg that the horse lifts the right leg. At the same time the body of the trainer pushes the croup of the horse over to the right. In the beginning the horse will put his right leg on the ground again. This does not matter, however, for this lesson is repeated until the horse understands the basics and leaves the right leg in the air for just a moment longer while the croup moves around. The horse is naturally praised expansively for this. The trainer continues in this manner until the horse can later on perform a quarter, the half and then a full circle on the forehand without putting his foot back on the ground. It goes without saying that this exercise should be repeated on both reins.

It is important always to look at the condition of the ground. The ground should be forgiving enough to make sure the horse's hoof can turn without becoming

stuck; in this way the trainer can prevent any possible tendon damage to the foot. To avoid the possibility of other injuries, the horse should not have studs in his shoes and the exercise should not be repeated too often.

I should at this point mention that there is another way to teach the horse this lesson, although I would like to oppose this technique. This is where the horse's leg is forcibly held up with the aid of a lunge line while the horse is driven sideways around the forehand with a whip. This tactic is dangerous for both the horse and the trainer and is more reminiscent of oppression than the fair and legitimate training of the horse. On top of that, two people are required; one to hold the lunge rein and the other to wield the whip that drives the horse around in the circle. I personally prefer the first variation.

SUMMARY OF TRAINING IN HAND ACCORDING TO THE IBERIAN SCHOOL

· *Refinement of the lessons learned, the piaffe, passage and the lateral gaits.*
· *Improvement of the bend and topline in the lateral gaits.*
· *To achieve a higher degree of collection in piaffe and passage.*
· *Development of the Spanish greeting.*
· *Development of the polka and the Spanish walk.*

Training
in Hand according to
the Viennese School

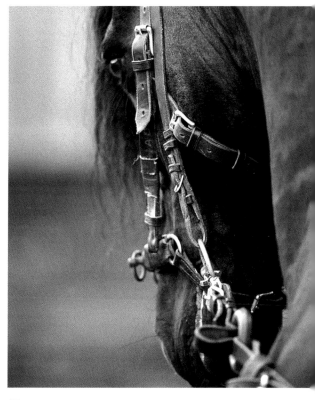

Training is simply called work in hand according to the Viennese school, and this work used in the Spanish Riding School is, like all the other techniques, an aid to help in the complete training of the horse. Exclusively used it is of no value and can even be harmful. No matter how much the work in hand has met with approval in the last century and how popular it remains to this day or even how many advantages it may have, its effect is often quite the opposite of that intended, when it is not done with the necessary knowledge and wisdom. The correct training in hand according to the Viennese school is, like the other methods of work in hand (with the except-ion perhaps of the work between the pillars), enormously tiring for the trainer at first. Nevertheless, if the training is applied in the procedure described, the trainer can

Viennese cavesson

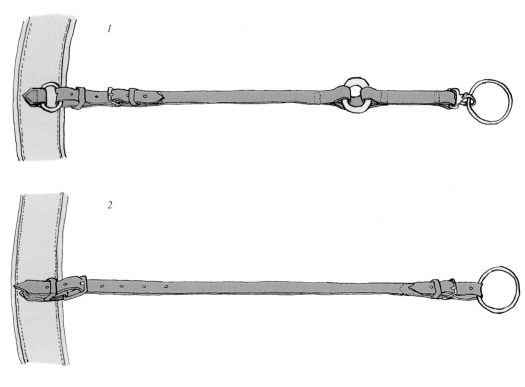

1. *Customary side reins*
2. *Side reins attached to the girth*

accomplish an unbelievable refinement of all the lessons.

It is, of course, always possible to use the work in hand for single elements and not only as part of the whole training system. At the beginning of this training it is important to keep an eye on maintaining the impulsion and even to amplify that, to employ that later in the high school movements, especially in the piaffe. The Viennese school offers the most thorough opportunity to refine a horse that is known today.

EQUIPMENT

The equipment for the Viennese work is nothing more than that needed for the work on the lunge, namely the bridle, cavesson, reins to lead, lungeing roller or saddle, side reins and lunge rein when necessary. The trainer needs to wear gloves just as before and to have whips of 130 centimetres and 200 centimetres in length.

PREPARATION EXERCISES

The horse is arranged to stand in the middle of the arena, dressed in bridle, cavesson, saddle (or roller) and side reins. It is best to have an arena with a wall or fence, for this will prevent the horse from falling out in the training. Much later, once the horse is more experienced in the work in hand and is capable of doing a correct piaffe in the middle of the arena, it will be acceptable to work in an arena with no side. The only time the horse is bridled with a double bridle is when he will be ridden in it after the work in hand. This should be the exception and not the rule; the snaffle bridle must be the bridle of choice. The cavesson is buckled in the manner described in the chapter on the lunge work. The choice of cavesson should suit the horse it is used on. If the horse is exceedingly sensitive, the trainer should use a soft, padded cavesson. If the horse is less susceptible, the trainer must use a harder, more severe cavesson on the horse. There is a lead rein attached to the cavesson on which the horse is led around.

At the start of the work the side reins are attached in a way that is not too loose but somewhat tighter than would usually be the case, for most horses want to raise their heads when they first start this work. But once the horse is used to this work, the normal attachment is used again. When the side reins are attached, the trainer should take great care that the horse does not panic, and this is also why the side reins are attached in the middle of the arena. The position of the trainer in relation to the horse is particularly important in the work in hand. In the ideal situation the trainer should be quite near the shoulder of the horse so that he can quickly get out of harm's way should the horse panic.

The trainer now takes the horse, leading it with the left hand, the whip in the right hand, to the track where the preparatory exercises are performed, those already known from the work in the Iberian manner: walk – halt, later on trot – walk and trot – halt. When the horse starts to trot the trainer should never pull on the lead rein. If the voice aids do not suffice, the whip is applied where the legs of the rider would normally be. When the horse wants to run ahead the trainer should apply a few definite half-halts on the lead rein and convince the horse to come back into a walk. The exercise is repeated once the horse is calmer. The trainer must also in this situation touch the horse all over its body with the whip, getting the horse accustomed to the feeling and making sure that there is no element of fear of the whip. If the horse gets a panic reaction again, the horse should never be punished, but instead the trainer should deliberate on whether the work in hand was started too early and the horse just feels out of his depth.

If this is the case, save the work in hand for a later point in time and meanwhile go the rider disintegrates, the work in hand should be put on the backburner until a later stage. The preparatory exercises of loosening and balancing the horse are similar to the tuning of musical instruments before a concert: instruments that are not tuned properly will not produce a good concert.

POINTS TO TAP ON THE HORSE

Once our four-legged scholar has successfully completed the preparatory exercises without agitation, he is ready to start shortening the trot. The trainer has much more freedom in the Viennese manner to tap the horse in specific areas. I would like to discuss this the classical points to touch in more detail:

1. **Front edge of the forearm:**
Increases action of the forearm and the shoulder with a horizontal or vertical canon (do not use when the horse can already perform the Spanish walk.)

2. **Back edge of the forearm:**
Increases action of the forearm with enhanced stretch of the leg (be careful with the Spanish walk)

3. **The same point as before, but tapping at the same time on both legs or the breastbone:**
The tapping of an extra whip at the hocks will cause a slight lift of the forehand, for the horse will pull the canon and hoof of

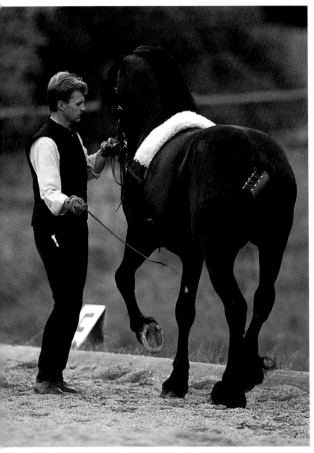

The trainer in the correct position for work in hand in the Viennese manner

back to strength-building work on the long reins, which will continue to have a gymnastic effect as well. A lack of impulsion and flexibility can be a cause of immaturity in the horse. Success or failure is, especially when it comes to the work according to the Viennese way, very dependent on sufficient impulsion. As we already know, impulsion is best developed on the long reins. If the ridden work under the hindleg closer to the forearm (will help tremendously with the levade later on).

4. Front edge of the canon on the foreleg:

High action of the canon when pulled back too much.

5. Front edge of the fetlock:

High action and more flexion of the fetlock

6. On the side of the stomach:

Overstep of the hindquarters, slight overstep of the forehand.

7. Under the stomach:

Forward movement of the horse; in some horses it will also help to get the hindlegs more under the body.

8. On the side of the hindquarters:

Overstepping in the forward movement while increasing the flexion of the hocks.

9. Back edge of the hindquarters:

Forward movement of the leg and increased flexion of the hocks.

10. Back edge of both sides of the hindquarters:

Simultaneous forward movement of the hindlegs through lowering the croup when hock flexion intensifies.

11. Side of the gaskin:

Overstepping with more action from the stifle joint.

12. Back edge of the gaskin:

 Lift and better placement of the leg with increased action from the stifle joint.

13. Back edge of the hind canon:

More pronounced action due to more flexion in the hocks.

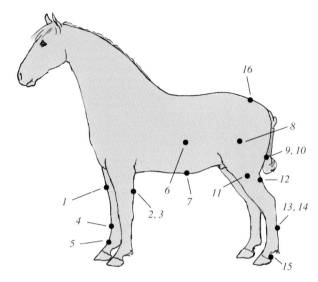

Points to tap on the horse

14. Both hind canons:

Forward placement of the hindlegs and more flexion in the hocks.

15. Between the fetlock and the bulb of the heel:

Forward placement of the hoof.

16. On top of the croup:

With some horses this will promote the lowering of the hindquarters; with very sensitive horses this will promote kicking out.

If the horse does not show the desired effect when the trainer uses the whip to tap the above-mentioned points, the horse is in all probability not ready for the work, physiologically or psychologically.

In such a situation the trainer must be patient until the horse understands the aids or the muscles are strong and supple enough to cope with the demands. Horses that are naturally "uphill" do not necessarily need the aids on the forehand, this natural lift of the forehand is normally enough to use the "motor" in the hindquarters. The trainer should therefore use the whip sparingly on the forehand and not work from front to back!

This horse is wearing a cavesson with a special lunge rein that allows the trainer more influence on the tempo

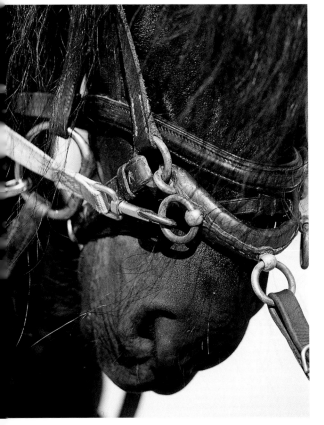

PIAFFE

When training the piaffe in the Viennese technique, it is often of value to have a helper to lead the horse forward on the cavesson. The helper should, however, never pull on the cavesson. The forward movement of the horse must come from the trainer, who is positioned slightly more to the rear. He taps the horse on the relevant points. The helper must only straighten the horse, either with the use of the lead rein on the cavesson in the inside direction of the arena or by softly pushing on the cheek with the hand that holds the lead rein. The helper must not move backwards otherwise he could have a fall, but move sideways, facing the horse. If the horse tends to run forward, the trainer can use a special lunge rein in the outside ring of the cavesson or the outside ring of the snaffle bit. This way the trainer can have an influence on the tempo and apply the necessary half-halts.

The horse starts off in a walk, the trainer requests a trot and then attempts the shortening of the trot with the aid of the tapping whip and the clicking tongue. The horse should then be given a pause to praise him on the one hand and on the other hand to get his strength back again. The same exercise is repeated and then the halt is requested and the horse praised.

The helper must move to almost in front of the horse if the halt is requested, this way he can start to understand the difference between the half-halt into trot and the half-halt into the full halt. It is espe-

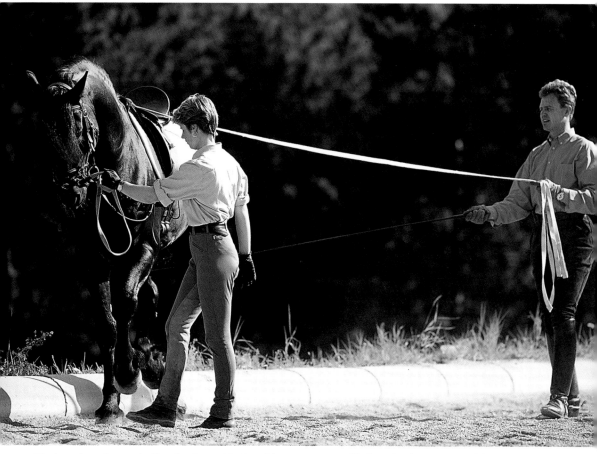

The horse has a lunge rein clipped to the outside ring of the cavesson to enable the trainer better to control the tempo.

cially important that the horse halts and is relaxed and stands quietly, which is not that easy to achieve in the beginning. Nervous and sensitive horses will often start dancing around when asked to halt. At first the trainer keeps the halt brief, gradually increasing the time later on. This restlessness should never be punished. To continue in the shortened trot, the helper steps back to the side of the horse, the trainer on the lunge rein clicks his tongue and with a delicate and electric touch of the whip urges the horse forward in energetic steps. The most significant part is to keep the horse's trust and never to underestimate the power a horse has: once the horse is aware of its power, the trainer will be practically helpless on the end of the rein.

This is the way the piaffe is taught in the Spanish Riding School. The downside to this technique is that nervous horses can the airs above the ground. In the Spanish Riding School the horses seldom develop problems with this way of training, for the Lipizzaners used there have very equable temperaments and tend to be more pliant.

The trot steps are now gradually shortened until the horse shows the first piaffe-like steps, while keeping the diagonal trot rhythm. As soon as the trot footfall is distorted, the trainer drives the horse forward. The change of rein is accomplished through a turn in the corner, where the helper changes by moving in front of the horse to be on the inside once again. If the trainer works with the special lunge rein, this is then attached to the opposite side of the horse. Obviously, our four-legged scholar is praised with every achievement. Incidentally, there is no bigger reward for the horse than when he is allowed to end the lesson after having done it with success. I will in fact regularly work my horses more than once a day for about ten minutes at a time, in particular when the horse does the work in hand. In the beginning the piaffe should only have a few steps and this should gradually be increased. It is crucial that the whip aids and the clicking of the tongue be decreased over time; the horse must be expected to perform the piaffe on a slight command and maintain it until the trainer asks for the exercise to stop.

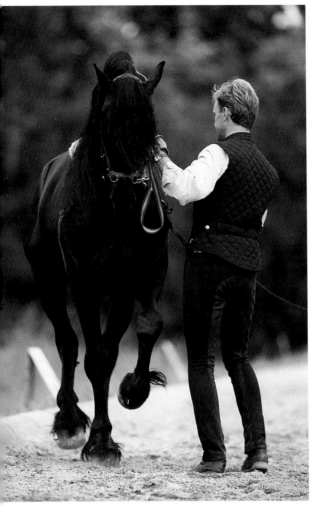

Friesian stallion Wiebe in piaffe in hand. The shoulder is fleetingly brought in as correction to straighten the horse

become especially anxious, which renders it almost impossible to continue the work in hand. For exactly this reason I prefer to make use of all the available options of working in hand that allows more forward movement to develop the piaffe. After this I will return to the technique of the Viennese school and refine the piaffe. From this the horse may be gifted enough to progress into

As soon as the horse is experienced enough in the piaffe to perform the steps lightly, the trainer does not need the special lunge

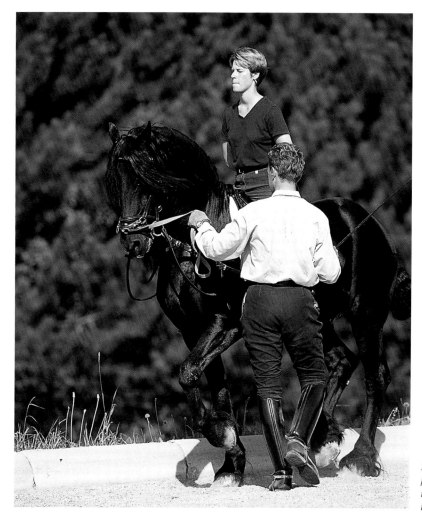

Piaffe under the passive rider: the perfect exercise to a better seat

rein any longer and can lead the horse on the lead rein attached to the cavesson and tap with the whip.

Now is about the time the horse can be burdened with the extra weight of a rider. The rider sits passively and gives no aids while the trainer requests the piaffe in hand from the horse as normal. This has two objectives, namely to school both the horse and the seat of the rider. Soon after the side reins are detached, the cavesson removed and the rider takes up the reins. The trainer continues the tap with the whip while the rider executes the piaffe on his own. In this scenario the aids must be kept to a minimum. In time the horse will be capable of commencing the piaffe with little encouragement and will maintain the piaffe almost by himself.

The horse must always be released back into the trot from the piaffe to preserve the impulsion and rhythm. While doing this, the horse is allowed to reach forward and down with his neck and the rider goes into rising trot. This is a valuable relaxation for the horse, especially in the transition phase between the work in hand and that under the rider. It goes without saying that this must be repeated on both reins.

As soon as the horse is proficient in doing 20 to 30 steps of piaffe, the trainer can initiate the development of the highest possible collection. This point will be reached at an earlier period if the preliminary work has been executed accurately. In the training in hand according to the Viennese school the Spanish walk and passage are obviously also taught and refined. The biggest advantage the Viennese method has over the Iberian technique, is the carriage the horse attains through the side reins, which place the horse in a specific outline while the Iberian trainer has to be the one in control of the outline all the time. The aid of a helper is usually indispensable, for the impulsion will disappear without the extra help. Impulsion and overstep can always be corrected and improved upon with the tapping of the whip while at the same time maintaining the action in the front.

AIRS ABOVE THE GROUND

The lessons for all the airs above the ground require on the one hand a horse with a special aptitude for the work and on the other hand a particularly well-schooled trainer. The lessons are developed in hand and later also performed ridden. The airs above the ground, together with the training on the shortened long reins, are the crowning glory of the art of working in hand. Nevertheless, I can only touch on the subject in this book, for the exact description of the manner of training would make this book burst at the seams. Furthermore, this training requires an enormously experienced trainer; it is for this reason that the riders of the Spanish Riding School do not become chief riders until they have managed to train a horse to this supreme level.

THE LEVADE

The levade is the deeper decline of the croup of the horse while at the same time lifting the forehand off the ground. The levade is developed out of the severely shortened piaffe, where the horse steps increasingly under its own body until the forehand actually lifts from the ground. The trainer requests the piaffe and with the tapping of the whip on the specific points increasingly asks the hindquarters to lower until the forehand becomes buoyant and the horse can actually carry his body weight on his hindlegs. The trainer now lifts his hand on

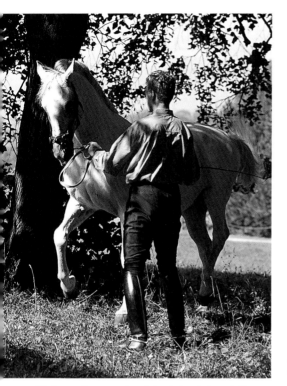

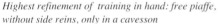

Highest refinement of training in hand: free piaffe, without side reins, only in a cavesson

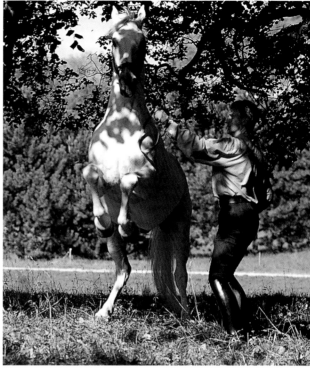

Levade

the lead rein as if he wants to raise the horse while at the same time bending his own knees. The moment the horse in fact levitates his forehand the whip stays quite still on the hindquarters, as a safeguard.

Do not ask too much at the beginning, for the levade is extremely exhausting. In a correct levade the horse will lift himself to an angle in the region of 30 to 35 degrees.

The slightest lift of the foreleg must be praised. If the hocks of the horse are clearly under the horse but for some reason he does not want to lift the forehand from the ground, it is possible to tap the horse on the front leg, on the back edge of the fore-

arm or under the breastbone. If the horse has understood the lesson of the levade but lets the lower leg hang, the trainer should tap the leg on the relevant points as well. If the horse does not lower his hocks sufficiently, the trainer should continue with work in the piaffe until the horse has developed enough strength and suppleness in the haunches. The quality of the lesson is reliant on the degree of bend in the hocks, which means the more the bend, the more the horse can place the hindlegs under his body and the better the quality of the levade. The other airs above the ground progress from this excellence.

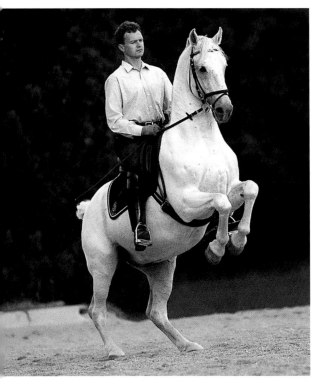

Maestoso Ancona under the author in levade.

The levade and the pesade, which will be described later on, are lessons in airs above the ground and have nothing to do with rearing that some horses are taught to perform. The levade especially is trained unhurriedly from the piaffe and is always a controlled movement.

When the levade is trained correctly, the horse will not use it as resistance, as is often the case in rearing. This is the reason why I never teach my horses to rear! The levade under the rider is initially also taught in hand. The trainer leads the horse and requests the levade under the passive weight of the rider. Once the hindquarters are strong enough and the levade in the

hand becomes natural, it should not present any considerable exertions.

THE MÉZAIR

The mézair is denoted as a levade with forward movement, where the horse performs a levade from the piaffe, touches down with the forehand and places the hindlegs even more under the body, goes up into a levade again and so forth. This lesson of airs above the ground can also be developed from the terre à terre once the horse has completely mastered the levade. The terre à terre is shortened so much that it eventually goes over into the mézair. In the earlier days the great masters implied that the mézair was the courbette, but today the courbette is a school jump, which will be discussed further on.

THE PESADE

The pesade is theoretically a preliminary exercise for the courbette (a number of jumps on the hindquarters). The horse raises himself on the command of the trainer still higher but, throughout, the hindlegs are stretched out more than in the levade. A horse that is practised in the pesade can hold the raised position for a relatively long time – I saw horses in Spain that could hold the pesade for up to 20 seconds. This is possible because the horses are in a much more upright position in the pesade. In contrast to the levade, where a great deal of collection is required, the pesade does not require such immense collection and there-

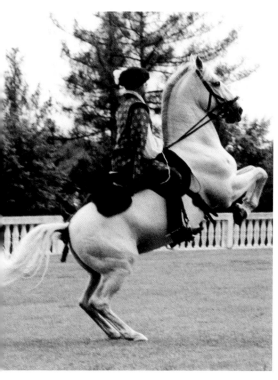

Pesade under the rider

seen up to fourteen jumps in hand - a truly amazing accomplishment! This lesson is also taught in hand first, the same as with all the lessons in the airs above the ground. In order to do this, at least three people are required. One controls the horse on the lead rein that is attached to the middle ring on the cavesson; this helper holds the horse straight. The second helper is behind the horse and controls the long reins that are attached to the two side rings of the cavesson. The third person stands next to the horse in the region of the croup and is in charge of the whip that is used to tap the horse at the exact moment for stepping under, hock flexion and the leap that follows all that. The long reins extend through the stirrups that are taken up and secured, to allow for a deep attachment.

The position of the trainer, whether holding the long reins or at the side of the horse with the whip, will depend on the situation. Having said that, the trainer must at all times keep his eye on the helpers, instructing and regulating them. It must be carefully taken into account that the horse is not necessarily used to three people working on him at the same time. For this reason it is a good suggestion to first walk around the school with the horse, halt every now and then and to praise the horse for good behaviour, gaining the trust of the animal in such a way. The next step is to request forward moving piaffe steps to make sure impulsion is maintained. The piaffe steps are then grad-

fore also does not need vast amounts of energy. In this stance the horse will need hardly any strength, but it is for the most part a balancing act.

THE COURBETTE

If a horse has an athletic disposition, the courbette can be developed from the levade by tapping the whip on the hindlegs. The courbette is a lesson in which the horse jumps forward on the hindlegs with big expressive leaps without ever touching the ground with the forelegs. Horses that are trained in this are expected to perform at least four distinct jumps, although I have

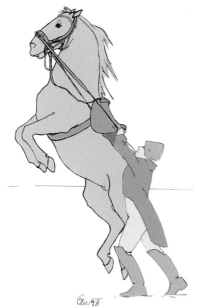

Courbette in hand

can link together three or four jumps.

Once the horse can manage all of the above without further problems, the trainer can handle the horse by himself and also manage the tapping with the whip at the same time. After some practice in hand the horse once more receives the passive rider. The aids the rider has to give for the courbette are as follows: the rider demands the piaffe, through tightly grasping the rein the levade is requested and together with this, a vigorous press with the legs and, when necessary, a tap with the whip will produce the jump. The rider must hold onto the reins during the jump to help the horse achieve the desired height and then give with the hand upon landing again. For a second jump, the aids are repeated. A proficient grip with the knee is of great importance in the courbette in order not to fall off the horse. If needs be it is better to hold onto the pommel of the saddle rather than to balance on the reins.

ually shortened and the horse is asked, with the long reins, to perform the levade. The long reins are held relatively low and taut, then the whip is applied under the hock joints, to prevent the horse from stepping back and to get the hindlegs level with each other. The person with the whip must now convince the horse with energetic, but not punishing, tapping and clicking of the tongue, to perform the jump.

If the horse actually performs a jump, the helper on the long rein must let the rein out into a much longer rein, in order not to obstruct the elevation. The helper on the long reins will demand a higher jump if the reins are held tighter, but the hand must be giving as soon as the horse lands again. When the horse is eager and shows no sign of resistance, the trainer can expect another jump until the horse

CAPRIOLE

In the capriole the horse jumps in the air from the piaffe, pauses in the air for a moment and kicks out with the hindlegs. The capriole is developed from the piaffe and the levade and is only performed with horses that are explosive and graceful. Once more a helper leads the horse on the lead rein on the side of the arena. The trainer moves on the inside of the horse with the whip, a special lunge rein attached to the outside of the cavesson. The horse is requested to perform the piaffe while the helper sees to it that the horse stays straight on the track.

The trainer regulates the tempo of the piaffe with the help of the special lunge rein and requests the levade through the half-halts and continuous shortening of the gait. As soon as the horse lifts into the levade, he is asked for the jump with the aid of a light tap of the whip on the abdomen and a click of the tongue, the lunge rein and lead rein must follow as applicable. A light hold on the lead rein will prevent the decline of the forehand. In this moment the naturally talented horse will automatically kick out to the back. If the horse does not kick out, the trainer convinces it to do so by tapping it close to the root of the tail with the whip. As a preliminary exercise the trainer can stroke the croup with the whip when the horse is standing still. The horse should on this light rap on the croup already kick out. This dangerous lesson will reveal the ancient force of "just" one horsepower.

Some important features in the assessment of the quality of the capriole is whether the horse jumps high enough to have adequate time to kick out behind, whether the horse's front legs are folded properly and whether the horse synchronises the kick with both hindlegs. The helper can later be omitted and the trainer allows the horse to jump on the lunge rein alone. Horses that are outstandingly talented for the capriole can later be expected to perform this under the rider as well. The habituation to the weight of the rider is much the same as when the horse is

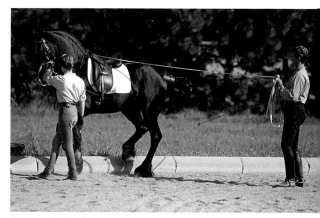

Preparation for the capriole

trained under the rider for the levade and courbette. The horse must be light on the reins before the capriole under the rider, the rider should never transfer his upper body forward, but keep it absolutely straight or lean slightly to the rear. The horse is requested to perform the levade from the piaffe and then, with the leg aid, to execute the jump. The reins must be taut in order to prevent the premature lowering of the forehand. At the highest point of the jump the kick with the hindlegs is requested with the rap of the whip on the croup.

The capriole with hanging front legs is considered faulty. A worse fault is the "standing" capriole, where the horse remains with the front legs on the ground and then kicks out. This is not part of the capriole in the classical sense and is simply a preliminary exercise to teach a horse to kick out.

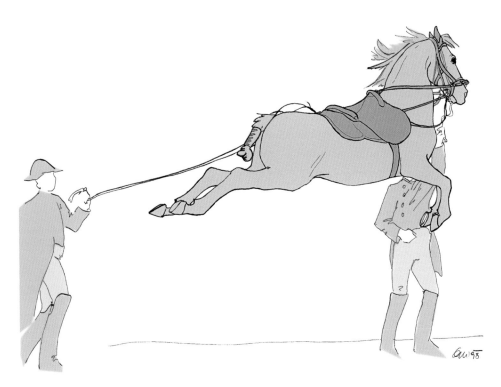

Capriole on the special lunge with a helper.

CROUPADE AND BALLOTADE
The croupade is the first step on the long
road to the capriole. The horse jumps in
the air as described before but does not
kick out with the hindlegs. Instead, he
pulls both hindlegs in under his body.
Because the horse's body is not horizontal,
the croupade can also serve as a preliminary exercise for the courbette, for the
horse clearly lands on the hindlegs. The
deeper the horse sits in the levade, the

higher the jump will be, for the entire
power of the hindquarters is used. However, the higher the horse jumps, the closer
he comes to the horizontal position.

In the ballotade the horse pulls his legs
in an extreme manner under his body. He
does not perform the kick though. Stallions that are trained in the capriole can
sometimes unintentionally perform the
ballotade instead. This is conversely no
reason to reprimand the horse.

THE SPANISH JUMP

This jump is seldom seen in the airs above the ground. It is not native to the classical school and is only mentioned here to complete the picture. This jump differs from the capriole because the horse has to stretch out the front legs as well. I have only once seen this jump, performed in Portugal, for it is very difficult to convince the horse to kick out with both the front and the hindlegs at the same time. This lesson belongs to the art of circus riding.

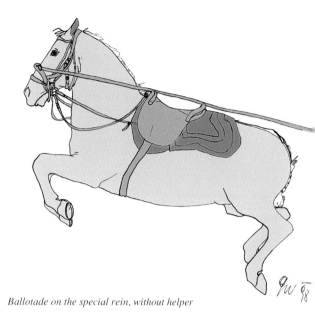

Ballotade on the special rein, without helper

SUMMARY OF TRAINING IN HAND ACCORDING TO THE VIENNESE SCHOOL

· *Accustom the horse to the work in hand with walk-halt and trot-walk transitions.*
  A helper that leads the horse while the trainer uses the whip
  from the special lunge rein.
· *Training in hand with a rider.*
· *Free work in the piaffe (trainer next to horse).*
· *Airs above the ground with the talented horse.*
· *Transition to the work between the pillars.*

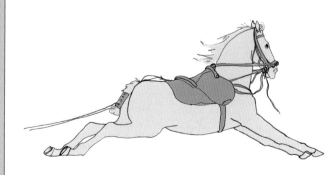

The Spanish jump

Work between the Pillars

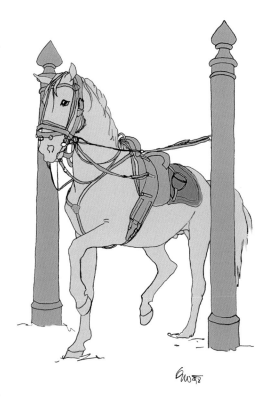

W ork between the pillars, as understood and studied by history's masters of the art of riding, is today found mainly in the Spanish Riding School of Vienna, the Real Escuela Andaluza del Arte Ecuestre in Jerez (Spain) and the Portuguese Riding School. The Cadre Noir in France still use the pillars, but merely to improve the seat of the rider. The inventor of the pillars is generally accepted to be, as has already been discussed, the French riding master Pluvinel. According to the latest research, however, the ancient Greeks used the pillars to work their horses. Eumenes, the defender of Capadocian fortress Nora, kept his horses moving by putting them in the pillars to trot.

The work between the pillars is exceptionally difficult, but nevertheless it is a superb way to further enhance the lessons of piaffe, terre à terre and the airs above the ground.

Dressed for work between the pillars. Pillars with metal rings, the kind that is found in the Spanish Riding School

His Excellency Herr von Holbein, the author of the Regulations of the Spanish Riding School, writes the following: „Work in the pillars should never result in a form of torture, which, in ignorant hands it can too easily become." Please take into consideration that not all horses are suited for work between the pillars and that this work can even be unsafe for the horse. Experience and a good understanding of the horse are essential for this work.

EQUIPMENT

The equipment required for work between the pillars involves by far the greatest expenditure when compared with other methods of work in hand. First there are the pillars: these are two columns that are arranged 140 to 160 centimetres apart. The best possible material for them is smooth varnished wood with a diameter of about 20 centimetres. The length should be 3 metres, about 1 metre of which is sunken in the ground. To prevent the columns from rotating in the ground, their construction should incorporate an appropriate underground component. The first ring is attached to the column at about 125 centimetres from the ground, and then another five rings should be added at intervals of 10 centimetres. The rings used must be made of steel or iron, with a diameter of 5.5-6 centimetres and 1 centimetre thickness. If the pillars are used without rings, a special headcollar is

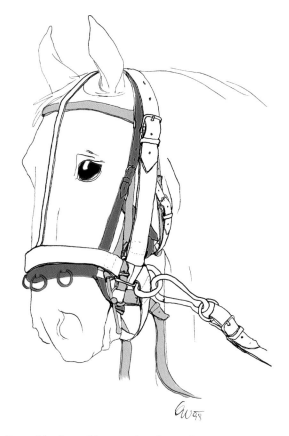

Dressed for the work between the pillars: pillar headcollar, cavesson, bridle with Fulmer bit.

required, made of rope where the ends of the rope can be tied around the pillars in a knot.

Another requirement is a pillar headcollar, made from rope or really thick leather. When a leather headcollar is used, it is attached to the pillars with particular pillar connectors that are hooked onto the pillars at the appropriate height by means of strong snap links. The pillar connectors are made of a double layer of leather or rope, are about 3 centimetres thick and 50 centimetres long.

The trainer will also require two whips: a driving whip and a shorter schooling whip that is, however, long enough to allow the trainer to stand beyond reach of the horse when it kicks out. In addition, the horse should be saddled and bridled in the same way as for the work in hand according to the Viennese school and have the side reins attached. Horses that are prone to brushing should be fitted both with brushing and overreach boots.

STEPS OF TRAINING

Once the horse has been sufficiently educated and is capable of performing the piaffe both in hand and under the rider without any difficulty, the trainer can commence with the training between the pillars. The advantage of work between the pillars is that the horse begins to lower his hindquarters even further while at the same time acquiring a higher lift in the forehand. The lifting power, especially that of the hocks, is notably increased, rendering the horse more powerful and supple throughout. To top it all, work between the pillars gives the trainer the opportunity to awaken any dormant talent the horse may have for airs above the ground.

When the horse is saddled, bridled and wearing a cavesson it is then attached between the pillars. The horse's tail is plaited into a tail holder or tied in a knot. As already mentioned, the work between the pillars demands understanding, considerable knowledge, exceptional patience and most of all a lot of time. If one of the above elements is missing, the work between the pillars can do more harm than good. The trainer starts with working the horse in hand to warm up the relevant muscles, then the horse is walked between the pillars to get the horse accustomed to them. Once the horse walks through the pillars from both sides without shying, the trainer asks the horse to halt between them and stand calmly for a few moments. The horse is then praised and the lesson ended. The whole event is repeated the next day. Once the horse is completely trusting of the new situation, the actual work can commence. Two helpers now come to the aid of the trainer and connect a lead rein on either side of the

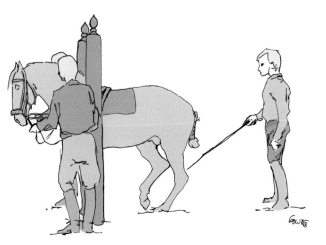

Commencing work in the pillars: "dancing steps" with two helpers

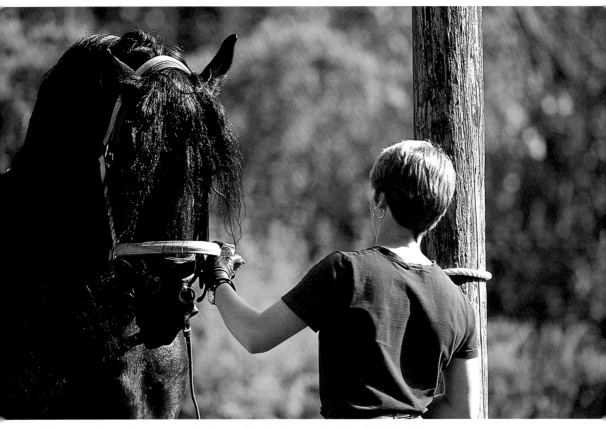

Due care and attention are essential when attaching the horse to the pillars for the first time.

cavesson. The horse is then quietly taken between the pillars by the two helpers. The horse is not yet attached to the pillars, but the helpers hold the horse on the lead reins on the left and the right side of the pillars.

If the horse becomes uneasy, the helpers lead the horse around the arena once more and carefully position him between the pillars again. The moment the horse can stand quietly and calmly between the pillars the real work can begin.

The helpers hold the horse between the pillars while the trainer asks the horse to step from one side to the other with his hindquarters. This step is called the "dancing steps" according to Pluvinel. This is a relatively easy exercise to accustom the horse to work between the pillars. In the beginning the trainer has to be satisfied with small movements forwards or to the side. Confrontation must be avoided at all times, for the horse will surely come out victorious. The horse should never feel threatened or oppressed, for then he is more likely to put all his power into resistance.

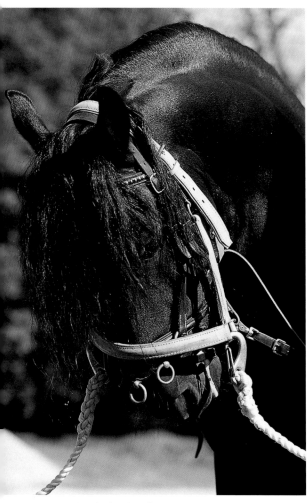

Attached to the pillars

attached to the ring in the middle of the cavesson with a helper holding the lead rein front of the horse to prevent him from backing up too much. The second helper stays next to the pillars to be able to intervene rapidly in any situation of panic if necessary. Consider carefully and weigh the odds before putting the horse between the pillars, for once the horse is fixed there is no possibility of releasing with the hand any more. The next step is to ask for the "dancing steps" while the horse is tied in the pillars. Another exercise that is beneficial to warm the horse up for his work between the pillars is the Iberian technique of the "goat on the mountain top". Once the horse manages this as well he is ready for the classical work between the pillars.

WORK IN PIAFFE

The trainer now commences with the work in the piaffe. The helper stands in front of the horse with the lead rein, which is attached to the middle ring of the cavesson, in the hand. It is important that the horse stays straight in these exercises so the trainer will, for example, touch the horse on the right side with the whip when the horse evades to that side while the helper places the head of the horse to the right. Once the horse is accustomed to the piaffe between the pillars in this way, the lead rein can be secured to the cheekpiece of the cavesson and the work repeated without the helper.

When the horse has been accustomed to the work over a long period of time, the trainer can carefully attach the horse to the connectors on the pillars. When the snap hooks are used to attach the horse to the pillars, the trainer should try to place the hooks on the rein without making any noise, for it is the noise that mostly will make the horse anxious. A lead rein stays

The trainer in this situation will step back, lift the whip and with a click of the tongue, ask the horse to perform the piaffe. The biggest advantage lies in the enormous freedom of movement the trainer has, to tap the horse on all the relevant points that have been described in the previous chapter for the work according to the Viennese school. If the steps become irregular or careless, the trainer can request the horse with definite taps to become more careful. The work between the pillars must always be interrupted with halts so the horse is not overworked. The disadvantage of work between the pillars also raises its head here, for the horses that have been taught the piaffe only between the pillars will have difficulty in making a transition into another gait. The result of work between the pillars should be a regulated, energetic and springy piaffe, where the horse lowers his hindquarters, lifts the forehand and pushes from the ground in a supple manner. It is advantageous to perform the piaffe without the pillars every now and again and to request appropriate transitions, full of impulsion in the course of action. Between the pillars, the piaffe or the airs above the ground can be given the indispensable finesse so that the horse is able to perform these lessons with the maximum amount of expression.

The trainer can also work with two whips, which are then utilised in the following manner: for example, the horse performs the piaffe diagonally with the correct amount of

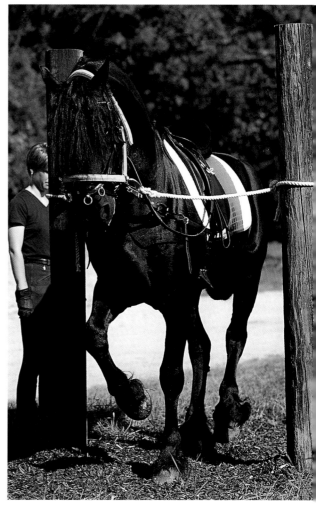

In the beginning a helper should be available to lend a calming hand if necessary

elasticity, but does not flex his hocks sufficiently, in other words he does not put his legs under his body properly and as a result does not elevate the forehand adequately.

The trainer now uses a driving whip as well as a schooling whip and asks with

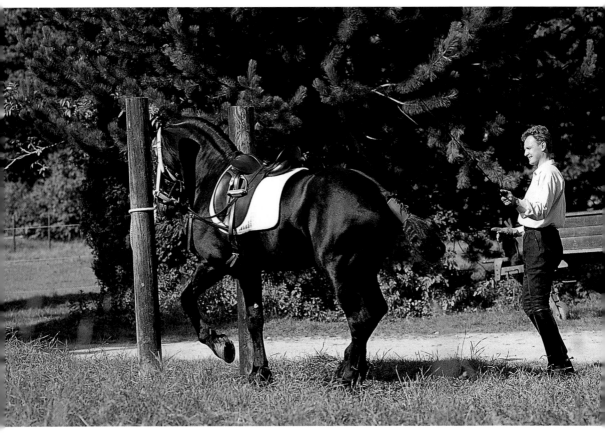

The trainer has more freedom to move around the horse in work between the pillars

the tapping aid on the croup with the driving whip that the horse lowers his croup, while at the same time tapping with the schooling whip between the fetlock and bulb of the heel shortly before the prevailing foot lifts from the ground. In this way the horse will place the foot further forward. If the horse kicks out or skips with the croup higher, the trainer can attempt the tapping on the thigh to see if the desired reaction is achieved.

THE LEVADE

Once the piaffe is visibly improved, the trainer can move on to the levade. As was the case with the work in hand, the whip is used to tap the horse's legs to move them increasingly under its centre of gravity until the forehand noticeably lifts. This is recognised by the fact that the horse will every now and again hold one leg in the air while barely putting the other to the ground.

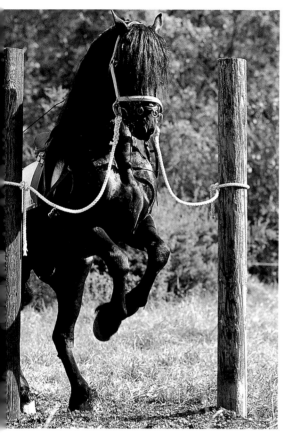

Wiebe shows his talent for airs above the ground

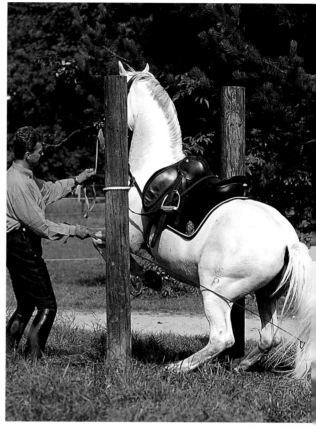

The first levade between the pillars

If the trainer now lightly taps the canon or breast bone, the horse will for a moment lift both his legs from the ground. When this is the case, the horse is extensively praised and the lesson between the pillars comes to an end for the day. Remember that the aids on the forehand are there only to assist the horse in understanding something better; the aids on the hindquarters are more imperative when it comes to the ways of the classical school. Without the relevant amount of collection, no levade is possible, for this is the highest degree of collection.

A faulty levade is also easily corrected between the pillars: for example, the horse performs the levade with the hindquarters well under its body, showing his talent for it, but leaves the front legs dangling. In this situation the trainer can softly rap the

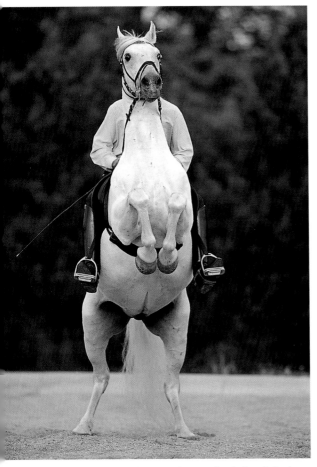

In this photo the original reason for the levade is clear: it hides the rider

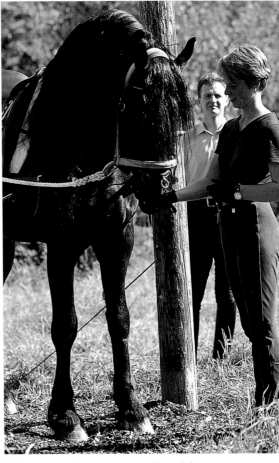

Praise is more than ever important in work between the pillars

canon with a bamboo rod to convince the horse to fold his legs further.

The trainer should take care not to frighten the horse with a forceful aid, for the horse will only place his feet on the ground again.

It is a wonderful phenomenon to request the airs above the ground between the pillars, but the trainer must be experienced and have an extraordinary gift for observation.

TERRE À TERRE

Apart from the piaffe and the levade, the terre à terre is another exercise that can be most effectively trained between the pillars. From the levade, both the upper thighs are tapped at the same time.

The horse will touch down with the forehand and jump with the hindlegs. Leave it at that the first time the horse performs the terre à terre, and end the lesson for the day. Little by little the trainer can ask for more jumps until the horse can perform a pure two-beat terre à terre with only the clicking of the tongue.

CAPRIOLE

If the trainer wants to, the capriole, where the horse kicks out to the back, can now be developed from the terre à terre by tapping the whip on the croup. This is carried out in the following way: the horse performs a terre à terre. The moment when the forehand is on the ground, the relevant point on the croup is tapped. This is normally sufficient to make the horse kick out, but when it is not the case, the lesson is repeated. When the lesson was successful, it is ended immediately. The development of the jumping capriole requires even more experience than is usually necessary for the work between the pillars. It is also important that the pillar reins are not attached too low on the pillars, for this will only result in the horse jumping into the head collar and using that as a prop. When horses jump in this way, they tend to develop a dislike for jumping and may decide not to jump at all. When cultivating the school jumps between the pillars – the highest form of art between the pillars – the trainer should approach it with the same care and respect that is necessary when performing this work in hand.

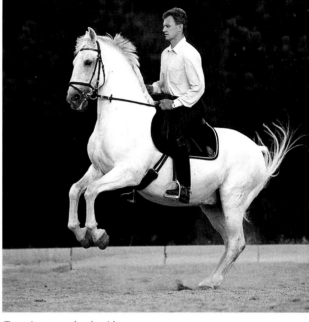

Terre à terre under the rider

SUMMARY OF WORK BETWEEN THE PILLARS

· *Getting the horse accustomed to the pillars with the aid of two helpers.*
· *Teaching the horse the "dancing steps" to familiarise the horse with being in the pillars.*
· *Attaching the horse to the pillars.*
· *Commencing the piaffe.*
· *Increasing the collection, cadence and power of the horse.*
· *Developing the school jumps in the pillars.*

Free Long Reins –
the Crowning Glory of Work in Hand

Work with free long reins is unique when compared with the other work in hand because it is an end in itself and not a means to an end. It portrays the final result, the maximum appearance of elegance that is possible in the training of horses. Without being close to the horse or without having any strong influence over the horse, the trainer can, at the merest hint, request all lessons that the horse is capable of performing to perfection under the rider. This requires a meticulously trained horse where the subtle aid has been the rule since the horse was a young animal. The ideal horse for this work on the free long reins must not be too big, for the trainer must be able to keep up with him and he must be absolutely trustworthy. The slightest indication from the horse that it might kick out towards the trainer, is a sign of a risk that should not be taken!

EQUIPMENT

The equipment for the free long reins comprises a snaffle bridle and the long reins themselves, of similar standing as that of the lunge rein. A bit with a minor lever action can be employed as an alternative to the normal snaffle bit, for example a Kimblewick. In the Spanish Riding School the bit most often used for this technique is the Fulmer.

The length of the reins needs to be tailored to the individual horse. In the beginning a lunge roller is also required to attach side reins to and these should be shorter rather then longer.

WORK ON THE FREE LONG REINS

In the beginning the trainer should start with an easy lesson such as the walk on a straight line, with the trainer walking on the inside of the horse. Corners, halt transitions and walk on free lines are the first steps. Both the horse and the trainer must get accustomed to the change of the rein across the back of the horse. The trainer lifts both hands over the back of the horse when he changes to the other side of the horse. This in itself can alarm the most sensitive horses at first, but should in general not cause a predicament for any length of time. If the horse remains somewhat suspicious, which should not be the case if it has been trained on long reins, the trainer asks a helper to lead the horse on a lead rein while he works on the free long reins. This difficulty should also disappear within a short time.

Once the horse does turns in the walk, for example volte, and is able to move on free lines, it is time for the trot work to begin. This is approached in the same manner as the walk. The trainer is at first satisfied with turns and long straight lines and later moves on to the shoulder in, which is performed in much the same way as on the long reins. The shoulder in is requested from a corner or when the horse comes out of a volte and the trainer moves on the inside of the horse next to the croup. The shoulder in is requested through half-halts

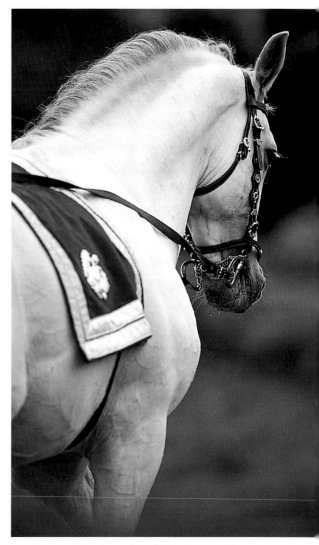

Another possible bit for work on the free long rein: the Kimblewick

on the outside rein, this is accompanied by an aid from the whip on the inside of the hock. As soon as the horse is comfortable with the shoulder in, the next lessons, namely the half pass and haunches in, can be demanded.

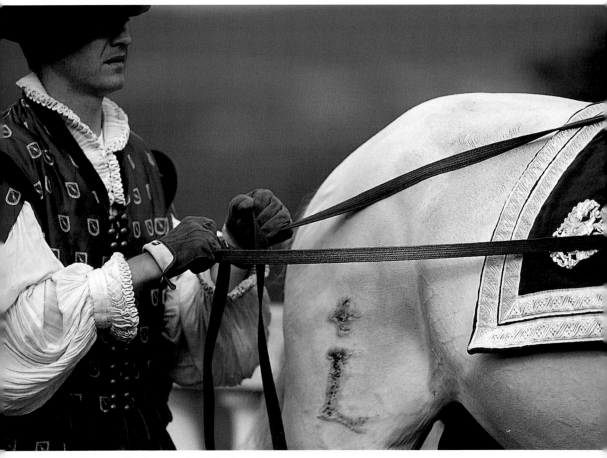

The correct hand carriage in the free long reins

When performing the haunches in, the trainer moves to the outside of the horse and also changes the reins to the outside. The horse is bent in the correct manner and the trainer gently drives the horse from the outside without losing the impulsion. The half pass is introduced in the same way, first the bend and the outline, then the half-halt on the outside rein, the trainer changes from the inside to the outside, the whip gently drives the horse on the outside and the horse will move into the half pass. When the half pass is established, the trainer demands zigzag half passes. The trainer asks for a trot on the left rein, changes direction on the midline, changes his own position and performs the half pass to the left.

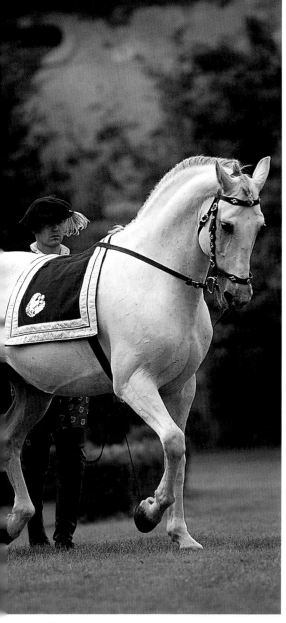

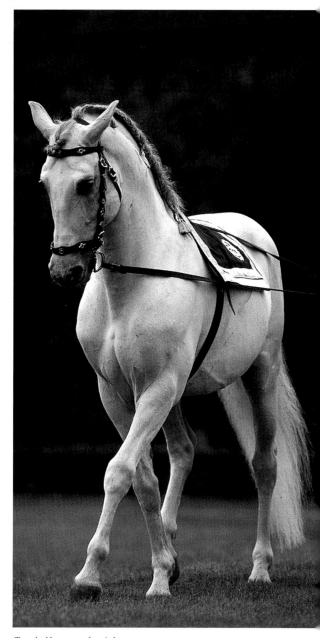

Renvers

Trot half pass to the right

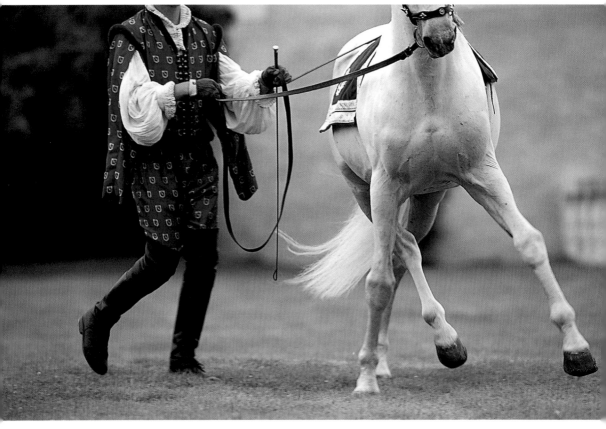

Dancing legs – tremendous cross over in the half pass

After a half-halt the trainer straightens the horse and bends it to the other side, moves to the other side of the horse himself and asks for a few half pass steps to the right. Depending on the skill of both the horse and the rider, this can then be repeated.

PIAFFE ON THE FREE LONG REINS

The trainer moves directly behind the horse in the piaffe, this means the trainer changes his position from the inside of the horse to directly behind the horse while the trot steps are gradually shortened. The trainer should take great care not to put the horse under too much pressure, for this pressure can easily escape in the form of a kick. As soon as the trainer notices such tension in the horse, he must let the horse trot forward to relax the state of affairs.

The levade can then also be developed from the piaffe; this is the only lesson in the airs above the ground that is shown on the free long reins.

PASSAGE ON THE FREE LONG REINS

The passage on the free long reins is often easier than under the rider, for the simple reason that there is no weight on the horse. This bestows added expression and lightness. The trainer asks the horse for piaffe at first, then allows it to win more and more ground until it is in the passage. The moment of suspension and the flexion of the hocks can be improved on by tapping the whip on the upper thigh of the horse. The trainer moves behind the horse in the passage as well, the only difference from the piaffe is that he stays one step further back so that he does not step on the bulbs of the heels of the horse.

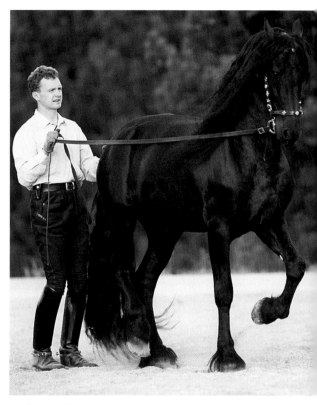

Wiebe in piaffe on the free long reins

CANTER ON THE FREE LONG REINS

Cartucho in passage

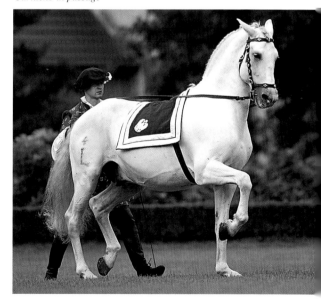

The easiest way to canter the horse on the free long reins is in the corner, with the aid of the voice and the whip that taps on the stomach or higher up on the shoulder. The precondition is, of course, that the horse is capable of a relatively short canter and the trainer brings an adequate amount of fitness with him! It is enormously important for the trainer to take long, giant steps and not run behind the horse in a hectic way that will serve only to irritate the horse. In the beginning the trainer moves on the inside of the horse and later, when the

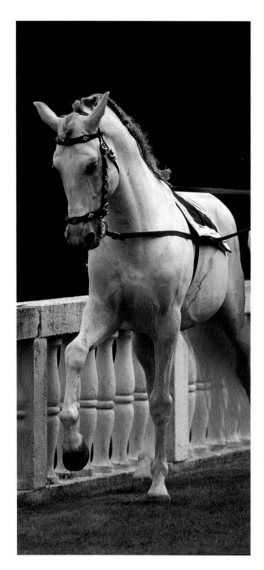

Canter on free long reins

horse allows it, the trainer can move on the outside of the horse in the canter.

Canter half passes are performed in the same way as the trot half pass, including the zigzag figures where the flying change can also be developed. The flying change is explained with the help of the voice and the whip aids. Once the horse has understood that, the aids can be refined to a mere half-halt on the outside rein. Then the horse can also be requested to start performing a series of changes as well.

THE SPANISH WALK ON THE FREE LONG REINS

The Spanish walk and the polka can also be performed on the free long reins. As is the case with all the lessons, it is not about teaching the horse the exercise, but rather the fine-tuning of the aids, for the horse should already be capable of performing the exercise. I always start with the Spanish greeting in the halt, which is where the horse lifts and extends the leg on the aid of the rein on the matching side. If the horse does not react, a long whip is used to tap the horse lightly in front. If this is successful the horse is asked to repeat that in the walk. If the horse has difficulty with this, a helper goes out in front with a whip held high. In a short time the horse will have no more difficulty with the Spanish walk on the free long reins.

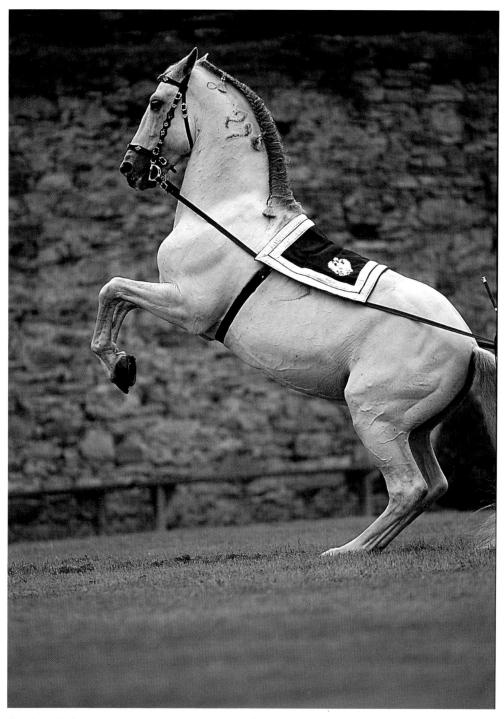

Pesade on the free long rein

Always remember that the work on the free long rein is not a method of training. It represents the final outcome of a long progression of training and makes a "complete" horse, which is already capable of performing all the exercises under the rider. This is purely to refine the aids of all the lessons. Another advantage is that the horse can be worked to an advanced age, even when the horse cannot be ridden any more. A horse that is used to being worked will need that to add significance in his life. When people go into retirement, they often deteriorate physically and psychologically if they feel that they have no aim in life. Well, the same thing happens with horses. I personally work my horses into a really advanced age and they are neither over-exerted nor do they have to relinquish their well-deserved respite in the paddock. I think that this is the true significance of the work on the free long reins.

Conclusion

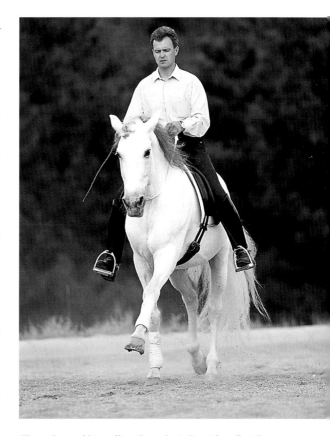

I have introduced you to a manner of training in this book that can enrich and complement riding; it could and should never replace it though. "Training the horse in Hand" offers a possibility to train and stimulate the horse without the interference of a rider's weight. As a conclusion I would like to elaborate on a few basic thoughts that accompany me in my life.

Why do we actually train horses? What gives us the right to ride on a living being that is not really made to be ridden? Too often the horse is locked in a stable for 23 hours a day and then taken out as an article used for sports, the rider oblivious to the character of the horse or what the horse actually does for the rider. In answer to this question one can only say that we do not really have any right to do this. The horse can never be ruled by man; we can and should only see horses as partners, treat them with the necessary respect and

The author and his stallion Cartucho in Spanish walk without a bridle: the epitome of mutual trust

admiration for the performance that they have given us.

Everywhere in history, where the footsteps of man are found, the hoof prints of the horse are found right next to them. The classical training of the horse, in which work in hand plays a considerable role, aspires to prolong the health of the horse and make life worth living, given that the horse is kept in an appropriate way. Love, patience, sensitivity and, above all, compassion should accompany our contact with horses. This is the very least we can offer our four-legged friends, who are willing to accompany us on such a long road.

Appendix

DIRECTORY OF THE HORSES SHOWN IN THE PHOTOGRAPHS

JULEPE

Julepe is a seven-year-old Andalusian (Pura Raza Espanola) stallion that I imported from Spain and is currently owned by my wife, Claudia. He is exceptionally talented and I am busy training him according to the classical high school. When he came to Austria as a five-year-old, he was insufficiently muscled and only schooled in the basic gaits. Now, two years on, not only is he very proficient in the basic gaits, but he is also capable of performing shoulder in, travers, half pass and Spanish walk. He has just embarked on piaffe, Spanish trot and flying change. His musculature has improved tremendously and it is all thanks to the correct riding and complementary work in hand that is suggested in this book.

WIEBE

Wiebe, a seven-year-old Friesian stallion from Holland with definite characteristics of his Iberian ancestors, is a light riding horse, which is not often found in this breed. He is enormously talented, has exceptional basic gaits, but was very anxious and suspicious when he came to me one and a half years ago. His training status was limited to walk and trot, of canter he knew nothing. He had no experience of side reins either. Today he has well developed muscles and has acquired excellent canter and lateral gaits, a superb Spanish walk and brilliant piaffe.

The classical art of riding and work in hand has given this stallion formidable confidence. He is now a positive horse full of expression.

MAESTOSO ANCONA

Maestoso Ancona is a seventeen-year-old stallion with many talented offspring that have been trained up to the level of airs above the ground. He has a strong character and requires a rider with ability to assert himself. His big talent is to perform a profound levade both in hand and under the rider in a superb manner.

GALIMENA

Galimena is five-year-old English thoroughbred mare with more scope than one would normally expect from a hot-blooded horse. I have been riding her for only a short while and she was very tense when I started with her. She has benefited tremendously from the work on the lunge and is now ready to progress to long reining. She is probably perfect for the work of Doma Vaquera. She will undergo a good basic training, like the other horses, until she moves on to the specialised work.

DON PEDRO

Don Pedro is a seven-year-old German gelding and a classical sport type. He was bought as a riding school horse and then came to me for training. He had several problems with his back that we now have under control. These problems return every now and again but are solved through specific gymnastic work in hand and under the rider. Don Pedro can perform lateral work in all gaits as well as flying changes. He has also started piaffe work according to the Viennese school and is showing promise.

CARTUCHO

Cartucho is a thirteen-year-old Lusitano stallion with outstanding characteristics and physical abilities, a really exceptional horse that does not cross your path every day; he actually found me. The first time I saw him, I was impressed by his charisma. He received his basic training in Portugal and was then sold to become a trekking horse. For some bizarre reason someone saw fit to teach this horse an extra gait called the rack.

He was ridden from Vienna to Paris and survived unscathed. I have owned him since he was eight. I have trained this horse in the classical way, following on again from his previous schooling and with the help of the complementary work in hand. It was hard work to re-establish his basic gaits, which have suffered as a result of the rack gait, but it has been worthwhile. This stallion can present all classical lessons, with the reins tied in the belt of the rider, or even without a bridle, as well as on free long reins.

Acknowledgements

The creation of this book is due to the many people as well as institutes who have made it possible to incorporate their knowledge in the form presented. I would like to thank everyone for his or her support. In the first place I would like to thank my wife, Claudia, who is an irreplaceable partner in my work, mainly through her calm and thoughtful manner. The superb Klaus-Jurgen Guni brought his professional and personal touch to the photographs, adding a significant contribution to the appreciation of this work. Working with him was a real pleasure for all of us! I would also like to thank the team Rosenberg in Waldviertel, Austria, especially the Hiebeler family, for their long friendship. They have allowed several of the photographs to be taken at their breathtakingly beautiful castle. Last but not least I would like to thank Brigitte Millan-Ruiz, the tireless critic of my manuscript, for the nights of endless toil to finally bring my ideas to fruition.